60
WAYS
TO LOWER YOUR

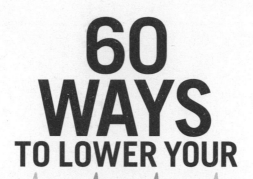

Blood
Pressure

ROBERT D. LESSLIE, MD

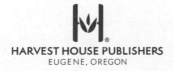

HARVEST HOUSE PUBLISHERS
EUGENE, OREGON

Cover by Koechel Peterson & Associates, Inc.

This book is not intended to take the place of sound professional medical advice. Neither the author nor the publisher assumes any liability for possible adverse consequences as a result of the information contained herein.

Unless otherwise noted, the stories in this book are fictitious accounts, used for illustration purposes only. Although based on the author's experiences, they are not meant to refer to any person, living or dead.

Unless otherwise indicated, all Scripture quotations are from the Holy Bible, New International Version®, NIV®. Copyright © 1973, 1978, 1984, 2011 by Biblica, Inc.® Used by permission. All rights reserved worldwide.

60 WAYS TO LOWER YOUR BLOOD PRESSURE
Copyright © 2015 Robert D. Lesslie, MD
Published by Harvest House Publishers
Eugene, Oregon 97402
www.harvesthousepublishers.com

Library of Congress Cataloging-in-Publication Data
    Lesslie, Robert D., 1951-
    60 ways to lower your blood pressure / Robert D. Lesslie, MD.
        pages cm
    ISBN 978-0-7369-6327-5 (pbk.)
    ISBN 978-0-7369-6328-2 (eBook)
    1. Blood pressure—Popular works. 2. Blood pressure—Treatment—Popular works. I. Title. II.
    Title: Sixty ways to lower your blood pressure.
    RC685.H8L46 2015
    616.1'32—dc23
                                                                2015021384

All rights reserved. No part of this publication may be reproduced, stored in a retrieval system, or transmitted in any form or by any means—electronic, mechanical, digital, photocopy, recording, or any other—except for brief quotations in printed reviews, without the prior permission of the publisher.

Printed in the United States of America

18 19 20 21 22 23 / BP-CD / 10 9 8 7 6 5 4 3

Contents

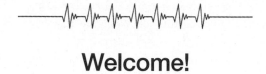

Welcome!

If you live long enough, somethin's gonna get ya.

Small comfort, but nonetheless true.

We're living longer now, years longer than our forefathers and mothers of just a few generations ago. That's a real blessing. But with that blessing comes some difficult challenges. Even if "our days may come to seventy years, or eighty, if our strength endures" (Psalm 90:10), most of us will experience health problems that weren't common a couple of centuries back. Various cancers, dementias, kidney diseases, arthritis, strokes, heart disease—it takes time to develop these things, and until fairly recently, we weren't getting old enough to experience them very often. But now we are, and we need to pay attention to how we live and to the things we do and don't do.

The way I look at it, each of us needs to give our self the best chance of enjoying good health for as long as we can. A lot of things remain out of our control: our genes, unforeseen accidents, and bad luck. But many factors affecting our health *are* within our control, and we need to pay attention to them.

You know the list. Proper diet, exercise, not smoking, getting a good night's sleep, knowing your blood sugar, cholesterol, and lipid numbers and keeping them in line, alcohol only in moderation, if at all. And, of course, there's the "silent killer"—high blood pressure. That's what we're going to tackle in this book. Before we go any further, do you know *your* blood pressure numbers? Do you know what's normal and desirable, and why it's important? Are you aware of the bad stuff that happens when your BP is sky high? We're going to explore those issues and many more. And we're going to stress accepting responsibility for and taking control of your health, including your blood pressure.

There's a lot of good news here. We *can* make sure that our pressure is normal and that we keep this silent killer at bay. It will require some effort, but you can get it done. Now's the time to take the important steps in assuring you give yourself the best chance to live as long and as well as you can.

Of course, our health and well-being is not wrapped up in our blood pressure, or any other measure for that matter. We are physical creatures to be sure, but we are also emotional and spiritual beings. It's all connected and tied together. We'll look at how that works and why balance is so important.

To get things started, it's time to meet Dave Jernigan. If you read *60 Ways to Lower Your Cholesterol*, you've already met him and his wife, Lisa. He's typical of many of my patients—maybe even you. He had to deal with his abnormal lipid levels, and he got that done. Now it seems his blood pressure is creeping up, something new to wrestle with.

Sound familiar? Let's find out.

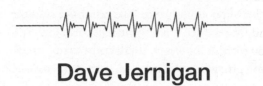

Dave Jernigan

"Okay, Doc, give me the bad news."

The forty-six-year-old sat on the edge of the exam table, his hands tucked under his dangling legs. He was alone this time.

"It's not all bad news, Dave." I tossed his chart on the countertop, pulled over the rolling stool, and sat down. "Your cholesterol is still in good shape, and you've lost a couple of pounds since you were last here. It's your blood pressure now that we have to work on."

"That's what I figured," he said. "Always something. As soon as you get one thing fixed, another pops up. Anyway, how bad is it?"

I appreciated his frustration with some of the challenges of getting older. Yet he hadn't had anything really bad happen to him, and he was in good health. It was my job to help him stay that way.

"The *silent killer,* don't you guys call it?" He managed a wry smile. "Slips up on you before you know it and then wham!"

"Yeah, this is serious business, Dave. Your blood pressure is 152 over 98. That puts you in the hypertensive category, but it's not dangerous. Not yet."

"What do you mean not yet? What's the worst that can happen? And when do I need to start worrying?"

"You don't want that kind of pressure hammering away at your brain and heart and kidneys, so we need to do something about it. But it's not at the point where something catastrophic is going to happen."

"Not today anyway. Right?" Dave leaned forward, his eyes unblinking. "Can we handle this with medication? A pill or something?"

When we had talked about his cholesterol and how to get it under control, he didn't like the idea of being on prescription medication every day, maybe for the rest of his life. He had wanted to try changing his diet and increasing his exercise to see if that would work. When it hadn't, he reluctantly started taking one of the statin drugs, and his lipids quickly improved. Now he wanted to jump straight to a pill.

"Dave, you're upset about this. Tell me about it."

He sighed and looked at the floor. "I have an uncle...had an uncle. Bradley was my father's brother. He lived out in Seattle and we used to go visit when I was growing up. He had this fishing boat, and we would go out on Lake Washington and spend hours, just the two of us, fishing and talking. I remember Aunt Sue would always get on him and remind him to take his medicine. He had high blood pressure and was on a couple of different pills. Uncle Bradley had been a three-letter athlete in high school and was always active, always in good health. Or at least I thought so. He didn't like having to take his medicine every day and most days he didn't. Aunt Sue would remind him, and he'd just wink at me and shake his head."

Another sigh. "Dad got a call from Aunt Sue one night, and we flew out the next morning to Seattle. Uncle Bradley had been working on his boat and collapsed on the dock. A stroke, the doctors said. Massive cerebral hemorrhage. His blood pressure was sky-high and...He was in the ICU for two weeks. Never opened his eyes, never said another word."

A silent moment passed. "I loved the guy, Doc. I was only twelve years old, but I promised myself that would never happen to me. That left a big hole in my heart, and I don't want to cause anybody that kind of pain. Not if I can help it. So, write me a prescription and let's get started."

"I understand what you're saying, Dave, but let's not rush into anything. Your blood pressure level has to be addressed, but it's not an emergency. If we can get it under control with some further lifestyle changes, you might not need to be on any medication. There are some things we can do, things that should be effective before we write that prescription."

"Okay, Doc, but let's get started sooner rather than later. What do I need to do?"

Dave Jernigan was motivated. Not everyone who comes to the office brings that essential factor with them. And many don't appreciate the risks and perils of the silent killer. Lucas Saunders didn't.

You Gotta Know Your Numbers

Just Barely

Lucas Saunders and his wife, April, walked through the triage hallway, following their nurse to room 5. He nodded as they passed me at the nurses' station. Fifty, maybe sixty years old, and he didn't seem to be in any distress.

The triage nurse handed his chart to the unit secretary. "Just some upper back pain from working out too much. Another New Year's resolution gone bad. He wanted to lose some weight and get in shape, but thinks he's overdone it." She turned and walked to the medicine room.

A few minutes later, I pulled the curtain of room 5 closed behind me. "Mr. Saunders, I'm Dr. Lesslie. What can we do for you this afternoon?"

He sat on the stretcher, legs hanging over the edge, and hunched his shoulders. "I must have pulled something in my upper back—between my shoulder blades. Started using some free weights a couple of weeks ago—flies, presses, that kind of thing."

"And he's done too much," his wife said from the corner of the room. "I told him to go slow, to take it easy. Rome wasn't built in a day and all that. But he wouldn't listen. He had a *target* and he was determined to reach it."

Lucas hunched his shoulders again. "I'm paying the price now. Hurts every time I move or take a deep breath. And it's getting worse."

"When did this start?" I walked to the counter and leaned against it.

"Not long after I started my new exercise routine. About three weeks ago. It was just achy at first, then started getting sharp."

"That was about the time we went to see Dr. Daniels, his chiropractor," April said. "He's a friend of ours and we thought he might be able to help."

I knew Bill Daniels and had sent him several patients through the years. He was good with musculoskeletal problems and knew when something needed to be passed on to an orthopedist or neurosurgeon.

"He helped at first," Lucas said. "Seemed to be getting better after a couple of treatments."

"But you didn't listen to him," April scolded. "He told you to back off the exercising until things were resolved, but you just kept at it."

Lucas shook his head. "Like I said, it was getting better, but then it seemed to flare up again and got worse."

"So that's what brings you to the ER today." I glanced at his record again. No fever, his pulse was normal at 76, but his blood pressure was elevated—160/100. He wasn't taking any medication. "Tell me about your blood pressure. Does it usually run this high?"

"The nurse said it was 160 over 100." April shook her head. "That's *good* for Lucas. It usually runs higher, but he won't do anything about it. His doctor wrote a prescription for some blood pressure medicine but he refused to have it filled. He said he could get it lower with exercise and losing some weight."

"No other medical problems, Mr. Saunders? You don't smoke or have diabetes or an elevated cholesterol level?"

"No, all that's fine. Just the blood pressure, but it's coming down. I think I can get it to normal if I can keep on losing some weight and continue exercising. That's why I need to get my back feeling better."

"Well, let's take a look at you and see what we can do."

I stood, took a step toward the stretcher, and for the first time noticed the large folder in his wife's hands. It looked like an X-ray jacket.

"Tell me about that," I pointed to the folder. "Are those your husband's X-rays?"

April held the folder out to me. "Yes, Dr. Daniels made these yesterday. He was concerned about a possible fracture in his spine from all the weight lifting, or maybe something going on in his ribs or lungs."

"Compression fracture was what he was worried about," Lucas added. "But he didn't see anything. Said the bones looked fine, but he wanted someone to take a look at me, since I wasn't getting any better."

"Getting *worse*," April said.

I took the X-ray folder, set it on the countertop, and examined Lucas Saunders. His lungs were clear and his heart rate was regular, with no extra sounds that might suggest longstanding high blood pressure. I had him stand and turn around, allowing me to palpate his back.

"This is where it hurts?" I kneaded the area between his shoulder blades—the rhomboid muscles—where most upper back strains occur.

"That's the spot, Doctor, but it doesn't hurt when you press on it—only when I move around."

"What about this morning when you were sitting still and you had the pain?" April reminded him. "You weren't moving around then. And what about the numbness in your right leg the other night?"

"That was just from sitting in a funny position," he said. "My leg must have gone to sleep. It was fine after I got up and moved around."

"How often has that happened?" I motioned for him to get back on the stretcher. "Is it numb now?"

"Just a couple of times, but only over the past few days or so. And it's fine now."

He lay on his back on the bed and I checked the pulses in his wrists and over his carotids. They were equal and normal. Then I checked his femoral pulses and my heart rate quickened. Nothing on the right, and maybe something faint on the left. His abdomen was soft, and I didn't feel any pulsing mass. But an aneurysm of his abdominal aorta wouldn't be causing his upper back pain.

I turned and grabbed the X-ray folder on the counter. "Let me take a look at this and I'll be right back."

Two nurses standing by the nurses' station looked up as I hurried past them to the X-ray viewing box and snapped the films into place.

My heart flew into my throat. It wasn't a compression fracture or a rib problem or something going on with his lungs. An angry aneurysm bulged in his thoracic aorta, threatening instant death should it suddenly rupture. There was probably some dissection of the artery itself, causing the lack of blood flow into his legs, and the numbness.

"We need an IV stat in room 5, pre-op labs, and type and cross for eight units of blood. And get the thoracic surgeon on the phone."

The nurses sprang into action, and I rushed back to room 5 and pulled the curtain open. Moments. That might be all we had.

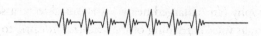

3

A Little (Uncomfortable) History

Hard Pulse Disease.

That's one of the earliest names for what we now know as hypertension—high blood pressure. Descriptive and accurate. Early physicians determined that if one of their patients had an abnormally strong and pounding pulse, they probably weren't going to do very well. And they didn't. The same is largely true today.

But when did we come to understand that this hard pulse was something bad? It seems the answer is thousands of years ago. Early Egyptian records indicate an awareness of this problem, and even had some common treatments for it. On the other side of the globe, Chinese practitioners observed the same findings and developed a whole field of medicine revolving around the study of the pulse—much of which exists to this day.

But it wasn't until the 1600s and 1700s that real progress was made in this area and in medicine in general. Physicians in England and Western Europe studied the complexities of the human circulatory system and began to develop an understanding of basic anatomy, followed by physiology (how various organs and systems work), and then pathology—what can go wrong. William Harvey was one of these gentlemen, as was Stephen Hales and later, Richard Bright. Many of the names of these early pioneers have been attached to common diseases that we see today. Bright studied the inflammatory conditions affecting the kidneys, with "Bright's disease" still used to describe a form of nephritis, the malady that ended the life of Wolfgang Amadeus Mozart.

In the mid-1700s it became possible to measure a person's blood pressure, using some crude instruments—prototypes of the meters we use today. Once this was doable, the concept of "high blood pressure" gained traction, and by the late 1800s, we began to figure a few things out. Cardiac hypertrophy (an "enlarged heart") was found to be associated with hypertension, as was "hardening of the arteries." It came to be generally appreciated that hard pulse disease—and by extension high blood pressure—was something bad that needed to be corrected. But how?

This is where things get interesting but a little uncomfortable. Today, we physicians are able to call on a wide array of blood tests, imaging (X-rays, CTs, and MRIs), and an ever-widening selection of medications when we treat our patients. Should we run out of options, we can always fall back to "I think it's time to send you to a specialist."

Such was not the case in the not-too-distant past. For hundreds of years—maybe a couple of thousand—the number one treatment physicians turned to was…bloodletting. *Cupping* was another frequently used term, probably because it was less intimidating. Belly pain? Let's take off a little blood. Gout? No problem. A liter or so should do it. Asthma? You get the picture. It seems the accepted philosophy in the medical profession was to *do* something. And since there weren't many somethings to choose from, bloodletting was the state-of-the-art treatment for a host of infirmities.

All of this raises the question of how much blood was appropriate to be drawn. I doubt that a person suffering with the ague or chilblains would present to the person doing the bloodletting a prescription for "half a cup please" or "remove one quart." Not an exact science. And apparently, if enough blood was removed to induce lightheadedness or even shock (which happened all too frequently), so much the better. It must be working.

In fact, that's why bloodletting was used in the treatment of "hard pulse disease," and even later, when we knew it as hypertension. If enough blood was removed from the circulatory system, cardiac output would fall and the pulse would become weaker. Something good must be happening. The problem was that our bodies make more blood under stress, intent on restoring the original volume in our blood vessels, and thus causing the return of the hard pulse.

And then we have our friend the leech. While slower in the removal of blood than simply cutting a vein, if enough of these critters were attached to a person's body, it was possible to remove enough blood to "balance the humors." They really didn't cause any complications (such as infection), and we have learned much from their many complex chemical substances—some of which include anticoagulant enzymes that researchers have utilized in a widening range of diseases.

Regarding the correct number of leeches to employ, it might have been a little like the recommended amount of daily prunes. Three enough? Five too many? But I'm sure there were guidelines to follow for certain diseases and complaints. And just so we know how common these were used, it seems that in the 1830s, the French imported more than forty million leeches each year for medical purposes. And you thought getting blood drawn for your annual exam was tough.

So when did we give up on cupping and leeches and reach for the prescription pad? That would be sometime in the middle of the last century. Some of the early drugs were quite effective in lowering blood pressure, at times to the point of shock and death. Several were abandoned until the development of hydralazine and reserpine, both still in use today.

Finally, and quite by accident, chlorothiazide was discovered. This was the first thiazide drug (what we now know as "water pills")—safe and effective and quickly becoming readily available. Not long after, the pharmaceutical landscape exploded, providing us with a wide range of choices for the treatment of hypertension.

But we need to be eternally grateful for the important legacy of our leeches.

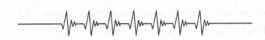

4

So What's the Big Deal?

"What's all this about the 'silent killer'? Sounds a little dramatic to me."

Dramatic? Maybe. But it's not possible to overstate the importance of hypertension and the destructive effects it can have on our bodies.

First, we need to remember that high blood pressure is very common, and it's the single most preventable risk factor for premature death around the globe. There are three important words in that sentence. *Preventable. Premature.* And *death.* That should be enough to get our attention.

Maybe not. As humans, we have an uncanny ability to rationalize our way out of difficult circumstances, to avoid facing reality, and to deflect uncomfortable information that comes our way. All of us should be aware by now of the health hazards of smoking. Cigarettes kill, and they do so without mercy or discrimination. Yet, when over sixteen hundred French people (of whom more than half were current or former smokers) were surveyed about the health risks of smoking, only half understood there was no safe amount of cigarettes that could be smoked daily. One third of this group thought that smoking up to ten cigarettes a day did not increase a person's risk for lung cancer. And more than half of the smokers were convinced they had no greater risk of developing cancer than nonsmokers.

What a great illustration of denial. And what a great example of the difficulty in motivating people to change habits that might be destroying their bodies.

We see the same thing in our medical office each and every day. But not just with smoking. A diagnosis of high blood pressure will frequently elicit the same nonchalant shrug and casual, "Everyone in my family has it, so what's the big deal?" Well, here's the big deal and why this is important.

Try for a moment to imagine a hammer pounding away at various parts of your body. If your blood pressure is elevated—at a level of 150/90 or greater—that's what's happening with each and every beat of your heart. Every moment. Every hour. Every day. As those numbers go up, the pounding gets worse, though you won't be able to feel it. But damage is being done.

Let's start with the heart itself. The constant strain of that hammering—being tasked with pushing blood through a high-pressure system—leads to enlargement of this muscle. This happens in the same way that lifting weights builds up your biceps or triceps, but in this instance, it's not a good thing. The left ventricle (the main pumping chamber) thickens and stiffens, which further limits its ability to function properly. This increases your risk of a heart attack or the development of heart failure (your heart can no longer keep up with the demands placed upon it), or even sudden cardiac death. We also know that hypertension is one of the causes of coronary artery disease, the narrowing of the blood vessels that supply the heart muscle itself. Less blood flow to the muscle, more demand. It's a vicious cycle leading to real problems, such as angina or ultimately that first (and maybe last) heart attack.

But what's happening downstream? What's going on in our arteries and smaller vessels? We want these to be as healthy as possible—the lining smooth and the walls flexible and elastic, yet strong. If our blood pressure is high, think about that hammer again, pounding away at those blood vessels. The cells that line our arteries can become damaged, beginning the process of *plaque* formation—the depositing of cholesterol and other unwanted things within the lining of the vessel. The walls become roughened and stiff ("hardening of the arteries") and these plaques can ulcerate, rupture, and cause strokes or a heart attack. This can happen anywhere we have arteries, limiting blood flow to vital areas including our kidneys, brains, and even the muscles of our arms and legs.

Something else can develop from that continuous pounding, and that's the weakening of the injured vessel wall. Much like a damaged water hose, the walls of the larger vessels can become thin and then balloon outward, forming an *aneurysm*. And just like a balloon, when that wall gets thin enough and that hammering strong enough, the vessel bursts.

This can happen without warning, and when the arteries in the brain are involved or the aorta ruptures, there's not much that can be done.

I mentioned our brains. This might be something we don't think about when we consider the dangers of hypertension. Aneurysms, sure. And we know that strokes can result from uncontrolled hypertension. Blood clots can form, cutting off flow to large areas of the brain. But there are other bad things going on, caused by that elevated blood pressure. The association between hypertension and dementia is becoming more apparent. In fact, managing high blood pressure is an important part of preventing and treating these devastating problems.

While Alzheimer's disease comes to mind when we mention dementia, there are other forms of this disease spectrum. Dementia refers to the development of problems with memory, thinking, speaking, vision, and moving, and one of the more common causes is called *vascular dementia*. As you might imagine, this results from a reduced blood flood to the brain caused by diseased and narrowed blood vessels. The main cause of these changes is high blood pressure. We are also aware of a transitional stage experienced before the full onset of dementia. This is called *mild cognitive impairment* and is also due to the damage caused by hypertension.

High blood pressure is one of the leading causes of kidney disease and failure. This happens in one of two ways. Either the vessels leading to the kidneys are damaged—possibly even forming an aneurysm in the renal artery—or by injury to the delicate vessels within the kidney itself. This leads to problems with the normal filtering of waste from our blood and the dangerous rise in some of these chemicals. When that hammering and pounding away at these highly efficient but vulnerable structures goes on long enough, the kidneys give up, stop working, and the only means of survival becomes dialysis or transplant. This is called the "silent killer" for good reason.

There are other problems associated with longstanding and untreated hypertension, such as gradual loss of vision and erectile dysfunction, but this should be enough to convince each of us that this indeed *is* a big deal.

If your healthcare provider informs you that your blood pressure is high and that something needs to be done about it, don't put your head in the sand. It might not be all that gets buried.

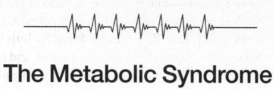

5

The Metabolic Syndrome

If you haven't heard of this, you probably will. In fact, you may have it. One in three of us do. *One in three.* That's a big number, especially when we consider the odds of dying from cancer (one in four), developing appendicitis during our lifetime (one in seven), or dying in an auto accident (one in seventy-five). And if the name doesn't sound serious enough, it wasn't very long ago that this was known as *Syndrome X.* In fact, the Aussies aptly call this CHAOS (**c**oronary artery disease, **h**ypertension, **a**therosclerosis, **o**besity, and **s**troke).

It turns out we've known about this for seventy or eighty years, and are learning more about *who* is affected and *how* we are affected. One thing for certain—this is real, and it has significant consequences. Those of us who bear this diagnosis have a significantly increased risk of developing cardiovascular disease (heart disease, strokes, and especially heart failure) and diabetes. Serious business. So how do I know if I have it?

Here's a list of five all-too-common medical conditions (all definitions are from the American Heart Association guidelines). If I have three of the five, I have the syndrome.

1. *Abdominal (central) obesity*—a waist circumference greater than 40 inches in men and 35 inches in women. Some experts describe this as "apple-shaped obesity," with adipose tissue accumulating mainly around the waist and trunk. We're not really sure why this is significant, but a

clear connection exists between this type of obesity and the development of several types of heart disease as well as diabetes.

2. *Elevated blood pressure*—blood pressure equal to or greater than 130/85 or use of medication for hypertension. A couple of important points here. This threshold level is a little higher than what we'll be talking about as being normal, and may be changed in the near future. The other point is "use of medication." More than a few of my patients have wrongly assumed that if they're taking blood pressure medicine, they no longer have hypertension. Nice try, but that's not the way it works. The same is true for those of us on medication for diabetes.

3. *Elevated fasting glucose*—equal to or greater than 100mg/dl or use of medication for diabetes. Here again, an elevated blood sugar or treatment for diabetes satisfies this definition. Some experts would include those of us with *impaired glucose tolerance*, frequently called *prediabetes*.

4. *Elevated triglycerides*—equal to or greater than 150mg/dl.

5. *Reduced HDL* (the good cholesterol)—less than 40mg/dl in men and 50 in women.

It takes only three out of five of these to qualify for the metabolic syndrome, and one in three Americans has it. These conditions are very common and negatively impact our health and threaten our enjoyment of living.

Causes of the Metabolic Syndrome

The causes of this disorder seem intuitively obvious. Some are just that, but others are more perplexing. While the exact mechanisms of this complex condition are not fully known, several interconnecting pathways shed light on its causes. Let's take a look.

Obesity (especially central obesity). This is a key feature of the syndrome, and a body mass index (BMI) of greater than 30 should alert a person and their healthcare provider to this problem. (For a brief definition of BMI and a handy calculator to determine your BMI, go to www.nhlbi.nih.gov/health/educational/lose_wt/BMI/bmicalc.htm.)

Interestingly, since only three of the five medical conditions are required for the diagnosis, it is possible to be of normal weight and still have the syndrome.

Stress. Surprised? This is complicated, and the association between the metabolic syndrome and stress is probably due to the effects of chronic stress on several hormonal activities in our brain. We know that stress increases cortisol levels (one of the stress hormones), which in turn raises glucose and insulin levels, increasing all the bad things they do. This may help explain the connection between psychosocial stress and the development of heart disease.

Sedentary lifestyle. Just what you would expect. Less physical activity is directly related to heart attacks and strokes, as well as to the development of diabetes. Many components of the metabolic syndrome are clearly associated with an inactive lifestyle. These include a reduced HDL, increased blood pressure and blood sugar, and obesity. We'll consider what constitutes a sedentary lifestyle a little later and look at appropriate types, levels, and duration of various physical activities.

Aging. Unfortunately, we're all a little older since we started this chapter. Not much to do about this, except be aware that the incidence of this syndrome increases with increasing age. The number begins to approach one out of every two of us as we pass the fifty-year mark. And more women are afflicted with this than men.

Diabetes. In addition to being one of the defining factors of this disorder, it seems the syndrome itself increases the likelihood of developing type 2 diabetes. We're not sure which is the cart and which is the horse here, but the two are clearly connected. The same appears to be true for coronary heart disease.

So, we know the importance of this problem, how to diagnose it, and some of the things that cause it. Now, how do we fix it?

The cornerstone of treatment is an honest appraisal of our lifestyle, identifying problems, and then making appropriate changes. Sounds simple enough. But as a physician (and sometimes patient), I can readily tell you it is not. Those changes will probably include increased levels of exercise, a proper diet (a significant reduction in carbohydrate intake is critically important here), adequate sleep, stress reduction (again, easier said than done), and carefully targeted medication. This is a challenging issue to manage, and one that needs to be attacked on a multitude of fronts. While daunting, it can be done.

When it comes to medication, knowing where to start can be tricky, and it requires some expertise on the part of your healthcare provider. Most of us—patients and physicians alike—want to jump in and get started *right now*. "Don't just stand there, *do* something!" The correct approach, as with many things in life, may in fact be, "Don't just do something, *stand* there." Or at least give some thought to your plan of action.

This is certainly true for dealing with the metabolic syndrome. We start with basic lifestyle changes, and then begin to attack specific problems with appropriately selected medications—sort of like a jigsaw puzzle. We start with the edges—something we can readily identify—and then look for other recognizable pieces. Pretty soon, the puzzle begins to make sense and things come together.

It's important to remember that we didn't develop the syndrome overnight, and it's not going to suddenly and magically go away. It takes a lot of effort on the part of the individual and a lot of support and guidance from our physician. But the results will be worth it—better control of our blood pressure, better control of our diabetes (maybe even eliminating the need for medication for these two conditions), better control of our weight, and reduced risk of a stroke or heart attack.

Who wouldn't want that?

6

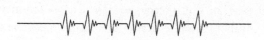

You're Not Alone

If you've been diagnosed with high blood pressure, don't feel like the Lone Ranger. Take a look around. You'll see another seventy-five million or so Americans with the same diagnosis. And as many as one billion people around the world. That's a lot. No wonder that hypertension is the number one chronic disease in this country.

Let's break those numbers down a little bit. Seventy-five million is a big number to wrap our heads around, but that's probably a conservative estimate. As we grow older, the prevalence of hypertension increases, thus adding this burden to an increasingly graying population. Some experts put that number as high as one in three US adults. When it comes to where and in whom this is happening, it seems the Southeastern US has the dubious distinction of having the greatest incidence (can't be the grits and fried green tomatoes). It is more common in African-Americans and less so in whites and Mexican-Americans. As with most bad things, men seem to be more afflicted with this than women.

When we look around the world, we see widely varying rates of high blood pressure, sometimes with a reversal of this male/female trend. For instance, in India, only 3 percent of men and 7 percent of women have this diagnosis. I wonder if this has something to do with the use of curry—something we'll look at later. In Poland (think kielbasa), 69 percent of men and 73 percent of women have hypertension. Fascinating stuff, and indicative of the importance of culture, diet, and ethnicity when it comes to this disease and many others.

As we noted, this is the most common chronic medical problem that brings people to their family physician. The American Heart Association has estimated the direct costs (doctor visits, medications, a growing multitude of tests) and indirect costs (lost wages, decreased productivity) now approach eighty billion dollars each year. That's a lot of money, and there's nothing in sight that would indicate the number might be going down. Just the opposite.

But there are some other important numbers we need to be aware of—and these are just as sobering, maybe more so.

We mentioned that the number of Americans with high blood pressure is at least seventy-five million. Of these, 82 percent are aware that they have the condition. That leaves 18 percent walking around with elevated pressures, oblivious to the danger and impending disaster. That's thirteen or fourteen million of us. All too often, the first inclination that we might have hypertension is when we have our first (sometimes last) stroke or heart attack. That doesn't need to happen, but those are the numbers. Significant efforts, some meeting with good success, have been made to educate the public and to provide for widespread blood pressure screening. More needs to be done, and we need to be creative and aggressive.

Then, of those 82 percent who are aware their blood pressures are elevated, only 75 percent are receiving treatment. That's a big gap. Five or six million of us know we have high blood pressure but choose to do nothing about it. To be fair, there are many obstacles to adequate treatment. Socioeconomic factors are important, with many of us not able to afford medication, pursue a healthy diet, or give up unhealthy things such as smoking or heavy alcohol use. This is another area where more can and needs to be done. We have to identify these obstacles and do what we can to eliminate them.

Here are a few avenues to pursue for assistance with the high cost of prescription medication:

Partnership for Prescription Assistance (www.pparx.org)
NeedyMeds (www.needymeds.org)
RxAssist (rxassist.org)
National Council on Aging, Center for Benefits (www.ncoa.org/
enhance-economic-security/center-for-benefits/prescriptions)
RxHope (www.rxhope.com)
RxOutreach (rxoutreach.org)

Lastly, of that group that knows they have hypertension and seeks treatment, only a little more than 53 percent ever reach their goal. Barely half. That's a concerning and depressing number. It means almost 50 percent of us being treated are not where we're supposed to be.

We can look at these numbers, throw our hands in the air, and accept it as the way it is. Or we can embrace this as a challenge, something that if effectively addressed has the potential to significantly improve the lives of many in our communities, and maybe even in our own homes.

But you gotta know your numbers. Then, if your blood pressure is high, you gotta do somethin' about it. And you gotta stay with it until it's where it needs to be. It can be done.

Take another look around you. One in three. You're not alone.

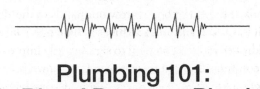

7

Plumbing 101:
Basic Blood Pressure Physiology

Don't freak out. You won't have to have majored in quantum physics to understand how blood moves around through our bodies and how blood pressure is generated. But after all, that's what this book is all about— understanding our blood pressure, why it's important, and making sure it stays under control. In order to do that, we'll need to grasp some basic principles. Let's start with a definition of *blood pressure (BP)*.

BP = Cardiac Output (CO) x Systemic Vascular Resistance (SVR)

While this may look a little complex, in reality it's an oversimplification of a group of intricate interactions. For our purposes, though, it provides us with a good framework to begin to understand what those numbers 120/80 really mean. First, there's our *cardiac output.* Just think of this as the amount of blood that's being pumped out of the heart in one minute. For an average-sized man, this would be about 5.6 liters or 1.5 gallons. It's a little less for a woman. This amount might go down at rest or way up with heavy physical exertion.

Next is the *systemic vascular resistance.* Think of this as the resistance to blood flow that has to be overcome in order to push blood through our circulatory systems. Sort of like blowing up a balloon. It takes a certain amount of air pressure to overcome the resistance of the rubber and expand the balloon. That's what your heart has to do with each beat—overcome the resistance in our arteries, capillaries, and veins and move blood through more than sixty thousand miles of vessels. That's right—sixty thousand miles.

But back to this formula. It's easy to see that if your cardiac output goes up and your systemic vascular resistance stays the same, your blood pressure will go up. On the other hand, if your SVR goes up and your CO stays the same, your blood pressure still goes up. It's the systemic vascular resistance that we're most concerned with, since this is the real battlefield in our fight against hypertension. When our heart has to pump against increased resistance, it undergoes strain and becomes enlarged—not a good thing. This strain is caused by the resistance of our blood vessels. The higher the resistance, the higher the arterial pressure has to be to overcome it and cause blood to flow.

This resistance is related to a couple of things. First is the size of the vessel (this is where our plumbing comes in). The larger the vessel, the lower the pressure within that vessel. As you would imagine, the opposite is also true. The length of the vessel also determines resistance (the longer the distance, the greater the pressure), as does the viscosity (thickness) of the blood. It's easier to push water than molasses through a pipe. And then there's the smoothness of the wall of the blood vessel itself. Cholesterol plaques cause roughening of the vessel surface, leading to turbulence in the bloodstream and more resistance.

Lastly, our bodies have been designed to adapt to a multitude of challenges. We are able to constrict our vessels through several mechanisms, causing the size or diameter to become smaller, resulting in an increased blood pressure. Adrenaline does a great job here. We're also able to dilate those vessels when we need to, increasing the vessel diameter and lowering our pressure. This is how nitroglycerin works. It's a potent vasodilator and lowers the pressure that a challenged heart has to beat against.

This gives us an idea of how we alter our blood pressures from moment to moment. There are both rapid, split-second responses—an increased heart rate or constricted blood vessels—and a slower, more gradual action—such as our kidneys lowering the volume of blood in our system or reducing its viscosity.

This is all really intricate and amazing stuff, and the regulation of our blood pressure is only one small part of our wonderfully interwoven bodies. Hard to imagine this all came together by chance.

Now that we have some understanding about how blood pressure is generated, how do we relate that to the numbers we're accustomed to dealing with? Let's use a normal pressure of 120/80 as an example. The 120 number represents the *systolic pressure*. This is the pressure pulse that the heart produces as it forces blood into the aorta, and if everything is working properly, this 120 is a good number. Part of the blood ejected during this pressure pulse (systole) stays within the distended arteries, and while the heart momentarily relaxes, this blood backs up against the closed valves of the heart. This represents the lower number, the *diastolic* part of our blood pressure, and occurs during diastole—the resting phase of the cardiac cycle. The pressure in our circulatory system never drops to zero (unless there's a real problem going on) and the diastolic number can be thought of as the resting pressure that our system has to deal with.

Now for a little perspective. What does this 120/80 number really look like? How much pressure does this represent and how much pressure can our hearts generate?

Once again, don't freak out. To make some meaningful comparisons here, we have to dust off our knowledge of the definition of *pounds per square inch* (psi). One psi is the amount of pressure generated by one pound of force being applied to an area of one square inch. For example, most of us are familiar with the standard automobile tire pressures—somewhere around 30 psi. But what does that look like? Let's start with millimeters of mercury 120 mm Hg indicates that this pressure is able to raise a column of mercury (much denser than water) 120 mm or 4.72 inches. A blood pressure of 180 would raise it 7.09 inches.

Okay, but what does that *feel* like? We mentioned the auto tire pressure of 30 psi. A soccer ball should be inflated to somewhere between 8.5 and 15.6 psi, while the pressure in a standard party balloon is around 1.4 psi. And our blood pressure of 120? That comes in at 2.32 psi. An elevated pressure of 180 would be 3.48 psi. That should give us some understanding or *feel* for the kind of pressure we have in our blood vessels and what 120/80 really means. And that's just about enough of flow mechanics and physics.

So we've seen how our blood pressure is generated, how it can change from moment-to-moment, and the amount of pressure or force we're dealing with. Now we need to look at how it's measured.

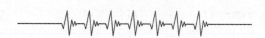

8

The Numbers:
What Do They Mean?

Now that we know how the pressure in our circulatory system is generated, we need to consider what those numbers mean for us, who decides when they're too high (or low), and when we should become concerned.

As a reminder, the numbers 120/80 refer to the height of a column of mercury, measured in millimeters, when a couple of important things are happening. The *systolic pressure* (120) corresponds to the peak pressure generated by the pumping action of our heart, while the *diastolic pressure* (80) is the minimum pressure in our vascular system while the heart is resting. Simple enough, but important to keep in mind.

We'll be talking a lot about "goal blood pressure"—the target level of these numbers for each person based on several unique and important factors. That may be a little different from the ideal pressure. Many experts will tell us that 120/80 is the ideal pressure for most of us—where we need to be living. But we're not exactly sure of this and the exact numbers that confer significantly reduced risk of a heart attack or stroke have not definitively been determined. As of this writing, though, 120/80 or less would be the "ideal blood pressure."

One thing we *do* know is that once we exceed a level of 140/90, bad things start to happen. Let's take a look at a chart that will help us with these numbers.

Blood Pressure Category	Systolic mm Hg (upper #)		Diastolic mm Hg (lower #)
Normal	less than 120	and	less than 80
Prehypertension	120 – 139	or	80 – 89
High Blood Pressure (Hypertension) Stage 1	140 – 159	or	90 – 99
High Blood Pressure (Hypertension) Stage 2	160 or higher	or	100 or higher
Hypertensive Crisis (Emergency care needed)	Higher than 180	or	Higher than 110

It might take a little getting used to, but these categories make a lot of sense. For instance, if your systolic blood pressure is between 140–159 *or* the diastolic is between 90–99, you fall in the "hypertension" category and will more than likely need medication. This would be "Stage 1 Hypertension," just so you know. The operative word in this definition is *or*. This is sometimes confusing for our patients, and also at times for physicians. Only *one* of the numbers—either the systolic or the diastolic—has to be in this range to qualify for Stage 1 hypertension. We need to be sure we understand that important point.

"Doc, my bottom number has always been fine, so I don't worry about that 170 part."

Well, you better start worrying, because I am.

The most problematic category is "Prehypertension." What are we to do with that? Is it possible to forestall full-blown hypertension? If you fit in this category, lifestyle changes need to be aggressively addressed (you'll see plenty of that in the following pages) and you need to monitor your BP more closely than if your pressure was 115/75. Most physicians would say no to medication at this point, but each individual's circumstance needs to be closely examined. For instance, if your pressure is 130/88 and your father died with a heart attack at age thirty-nine or your mother with a stroke at forty-two, your doctor might want to get your BP below 120/80 and keep it there. For most of us, though, lifestyle changes should be the first line of attack, and for many, this will be successful.

It's safe to say that the lower the blood pressure the better, as long as that low blood pressure doesn't cause symptoms such as dizziness, weakness, or fatigue. If you had to pick a perfect set of numbers, it would be a 110/70 with a heart rate of 55.

I disagree with one of the guidelines from the AHA, specifically the "Hypertensive Crisis" category and the admonition to seek emergency care. During my twenty-five years in the ER, you might think I've seen my share of people coming in with sky-high blood pressures, and you'd be right. Let's use 190/112 as an example. Oh, and *you* get to be the ER doc.

John M., a forty-five-year-old insurance salesman, comes to the ER after injuring his right ankle playing basketball. His ankle is swollen, tender, and his blood pressure is 190/112. No history of hypertension and no medications. He doesn't smoke, and your examination indicates no evidence of heart disease, kidney disease, or any mental impairment or neurological complaints. What do you do?

- Strap him down and draw off a liter of blood.

- Start an IV and give him oxygen through some nasal prongs.

- Direct the nurse to give him nitroglycerin under his tongue.

- Start some high-powered IV medication to get his pressure under 150/90 as quickly as you can.

- None of the above.

And then there's Sally J, a forty-three-year-old banking executive who presents to the ER complaining of the gradual onset of a dull headache over the past few days. It just won't go away, even with over-the-counter medications. Her blood pressure is 190/112, and though she's alert, she is clearly uncomfortable with this headache. While in the ER, she develops nausea and vomits once. She's on no medication and has no history of any significant medical problems. What do you do? She's not going to let you strap her down and draw off any blood.

- Start an IV, draw labs, and get an EKG.

- Give her high-powered medication to lower her pressure to normal over the next twenty minutes.

- Give her something for her headache, wait thirty minutes,

and see if it goes away. If it does and her nausea is better, she can go home.

* Begin blood pressure treatment, with a goal of gradually lowering it over the next several hours. Find a bed for her upstairs.

* None of the above.

Okay, what do you think? With John M., the correct plan of treatment would be to do none of the above. After you've ruled out any "target organ damage" (heart, kidneys, brain), you should address the reason he's in the ER, consider starting him on some blood pressure medication, and impress upon him the importance of seeing his primary care physician in the next few days. He most certainly will have hypertension, but he's probably been walking around at this level for a while. He doesn't need to be given high-powered medication in the ER—something that might cause more harm than good. The key here is that he doesn't have any evidence of significant changes from his hypertension. It's safe to send him home with assurances of close follow-up.

Sally J. presents a different problem. She *does* have potential target organ damage (her unrelenting headache and vomiting) and will need immediate evaluation, such as an MRI of her brain. After starting an IV, getting an EKG, and checking labs, her pressure needs to be lowered gradually, understanding that a precipitous drop could cause some real problems.

Two identical blood pressures, two different people, two different interventions. Something to keep in mind should you or a loved one find yourselves in this circumstance.

So back to those numbers—our systolic and diastolic pressures. We've got an understanding of where they should be. Now let's take a look at how we measure them.

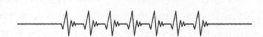

9

Measuring Your Blood Pressure: Is There a Right Way?

The answer is yes. There is a right way to measure your BP. And there's a wrong way. In fact, there are *several* wrong ways. Here are some thoughts based on what the folks at the National Institutes of Health (NIH) have to say about this.

Your blood pressure should be measured while sitting, legs uncrossed and feet on the floor. Sleeves should be rolled up so that your arm is bare. Your arm should be supported so that the upper arm is at or near heart level. The cuff should be placed snugly, with the lower edge of the cuff one inch above your elbow.

The size of the cuff is important, since one that is too small can give a falsely high reading, while a cuff that's too large can miss an elevated blood pressure. A good rule of thumb is that the cuff should cover two-thirds of the arm—from elbow to shoulder. Another general rule, though harder to determine, is that the inflatable part of the cuff should cover about 80 percent of the *circumference* of the upper arm. We need to pay attention to this, because the proper sizing of the cuff does make a difference. If you have a concern, voice it to the person taking your pressure or to your physician. We're all interested in getting the most accurate measurement possible.

Once in place, the cuff should be inflated quickly. You're going to feel some tightness, which is just a part of the process. If you feel pain, that's probably too much pressure and shouldn't happen.

Once inflated, the valve on the cuff should be slowly opened, allowing the pressure to gradually fall. This gradual *deflation* is critical and should take as long as ten to fifteen seconds. The more gradual the release the better, especially if your heart rate is slow. If you release the pressure too fast, you're just not going to hear enough beats to get an accurate reading. You need to pay attention here. Several years ago, an inexperienced ER tech routinely took the blood pressures of most of the patients coming through the triage area. I thought it peculiar that almost all of her patients had BPs of 120/80, and one day I decided to watch her technique. She used the right-sized cuff, placed it properly on the arm, held the bell of her stethoscope correctly over the artery at the elbow, then rapidly inflated the cuff. The problem became apparent as I watched her quickly open the valve and deflate the cuff in two or three seconds. There was no way she could hear more than a couple of heartbeats, much less determine an accurate pressure. It was time for some remedial education and training.

Two, maybe three times is the max for taking a blood pressure in the same arm at one setting, with each reading being at least one minute apart.

A couple of pointers to ensure an accurate measurement:

- Don't smoke thirty minutes before entering the office. In fact, don't smoke at all.

- Rest quietly at least five minutes before your BP is taken.

- Don't have your pressure taken if you're experiencing undue stress. Yes, bad traffic before getting to the office or an argument with your spouse or child or boss can make your pressure go up.

- It's probably reasonable to avoid caffeine for thirty minutes before measuring.

- If you're taking your BP at home, note the time of day. Our blood pressures vary during the day-night cycle, with lower pressures occurring in the morning more than in the evening. It may also be higher while we're at work, and it's lowest while we're sleeping.

So, now you know the proper technique to ensure an accurate blood pressure reading, whether someone does it for you or you're measuring it at home. The important thing is to get it measured. There are three places where this can happen: your physician's office, your home, or continuous measuring for twelve to twenty-four hours with a process called *ambulatory blood pressure monitoring*. (You'll notice I left out grocery stores, drugstores, and any other locations where self-monitoring BP machines might be located. Remember, one size cuff doesn't fit all, thus potentially leading to an erroneous measurement. And there will always be the question of standardization and routine calibration, not to mention a potentially crowded, loud, and stressful environment.)

There are some significant differences between these three places, with one of them clearly standing out as the gold standard. Let's take a look at what we're talking about.

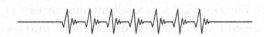

10

Office-Based Blood Pressure Management

"Mr. Jones, have a seat and roll up your sleeve."

The office or clinic setting has historically been the site where blood pressure readings and management occurs. That's probably not going to change anytime soon. In fact, the blood pressure readings used in almost all of the large hypertension studies have been done in medical offices. However, there are a couple of problems.

The goal is always to get the most accurate reading possible. If we assume that we have a good blood pressure monitor at home and that we're using the proper techniques discussed in the last chapter, office-based readings may not be as accurate as those taken at home.

"But I thought the office BP was the gold standard. Why wouldn't it be?"

First, let's presume that the proper technique is being used in the office. This may be a big presumption, depending on the experience and momentary focus of the person taking the measurement. Automated devices are helpful in this regard, removing much of the potential for human error. They are more accurate and consistent than manual methods. The cost is significant, though, and many medical practices can't or won't make the financial commitment for these machines.

But regardless of the method of measurement being used, this reading represents a snapshot—a very limited picture of what your blood pressure is doing throughout the day. A normal reading doesn't necessarily mean you don't have hypertension, and a single high reading doesn't mean you need to be started on medication. Here are some reasons this can become difficult.

The time of day your BP is measured is very important. Our blood pressures vary and can change from hour to hour, even from moment to moment. It will usually be lowest while sleeping and in the morning, then higher in the afternoon. Making this more complex is that several factors can affect our pressures while in the office. White-coat syndrome is real, and is one of these factors. Mental and emotional stress as well as recent physical activity (such as rushing from your car to make it in time for your appointment) can raise your blood pressure.

Caffeine can rapidly (though briefly) elevate your blood pressure, especially if you're not used to consuming it. Coffee and tea immediately come to mind, but soft drinks and energy beverages can be loaded with this stimulant as well.

Exposure to a cold environment (winter weather or a chilly waiting room) can raise your BP as much as 10 mm Hg. This usually doesn't happen above a temperature of fifty-five degrees or so.

We know that smoking can raise our BP and that this effect can last as long as thirty minutes. You've seen it (maybe *done* it)—that last deep drag before entering the waiting room. Depending on the time frame, this can elevate your pressure by 10–15 mmHg.

So it's easy to see how that one snapshot can be misleading. But for most of us, that's how our blood pressure is measured, and if we're diagnosed with hypertension, that's how it's managed—in the office or clinic.

What are some things we can do to ensure the most accurate reading in the office?

Don't drink or smoke within half an hour (preferably at least an hour) before coming for your appointment.

If at all possible, avoid stressful situations (let me know how to do this one!) and use whatever time you have in the waiting or exam room to calm yourself. This emotional aspect of our BP fluctuations turns out to be significant.

Have your BP checked in the office at about the same time for each visit, if possible. This is not as critical as some of the other points, but could catch your pressure while it's up or down, depending on the time of day, and potentially be misleading.

Lastly, most experts don't want us to take our BP medications *before* the office visit. This allows for a more precise measurement of our lowest level without medicine and helps our physician determine the effectiveness (or lack thereof) of our treatment and control. This would mean not taking our morning dose on the day of our appointment. Some people get a little nervous when instructed to do this, especially if their visit is not scheduled until the afternoon. The ideal strategy would be to have our measurements taken at nine in the morning, not having taking our medication and maybe not having eaten anything. That's usually not going to be feasible. So what are we to do? Is there a better way of following our blood pressures and managing this problem?

The answer is yes. Let's take a look at two other options, both of which are more accurate than going to your doctor's office.

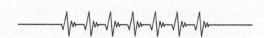

11

Home Blood Pressure Monitoring: Is It a Waste of Time?

"Doc, I've been checking my blood pressure at home for years now, but my sister tells me I'm just wasting my time. She says those machines aren't any good and you don't pay any attention to the readings anyway. What gives here?"

What gives? Plenty.

First, your sister is all wrong about this. Home blood pressure readings, if done correctly, can be just as accurate and useful—probably more so—than those taken in the office. And yes, we pay attention to those readings. Or at least we should. We know that properly taken pressures at home will give us a truer picture of a person's BP, much more meaningful than a single measurement taken in a sometimes hectic doctor's office.

Almost every study that compares office versus home readings finds consistently lower blood pressure when this vital sign is measured away from the clinic. This is important, since while we don't want to miss the diagnosis of hypertension, we also don't want to mislabel an individual as being hypertensive and have them on unnecessary medication. (And maybe paying higher health insurance premiums.)

But what's the best routine if you're going to do this? How often and when should we be measuring our pressures at home? The answer's not clear-cut, but most physicians recommend at least three or four readings a day if you're trying to determine your baseline pressure. The time of day needs to be noted with each reading, and the measurements need to be spread out. As a physician, I'd like to see a dozen or so of these readings. That gives me some good information and something I can deal with.

If you have an established history of hypertension and are on medication, it's reasonable to check your pressure every couple of days, assuming it is now in the normal range. If you're just starting treatment, two readings a day—one in the morning and one in the evening—should suffice. We'll talk about balance later on, but this is one of those areas where we don't want to become obsessed with inflating that cuff every couple of hours, or with every instance of not feeling well, or just because your spouse remarks upon your flushed face.

Every once in a while, a well-intended patient will come into the office with a notebook full of BP readings. On one occasion, I was handed a notepad loaded with dates and numbers. Upon closer inspection, I noted that some of these blood pressure readings were spaced only ten to fifteen minutes apart. I felt as if I was studying a vital sign flow sheet in the ICU. Balance. You and your healthcare provider can map out a reasonable strategy and then just stick with it.

"Okay, so I should be checking my blood pressure at home. What kind of thing do I buy, where can I get it, and how much is it gonna cost me?"

Let's start with the "kind of thing." I have no financial interest in any of the following recommendations. (The only kickback I've ever gotten was from trying to snuggle with my wife.) In researching this, I gathered the best information I could find—including the ratings of these devices by one of our highly regarded consumer publications—and will present a couple of viable options. You can do your own research, ask your friends, and draw your own conclusions.

I was able to find four home monitors that were consistently highly rated on accuracy and convenience-of-use.

- Omron 10 series BP786
- iHealth Dock BP3
- A&D Medical UA767F
- Rite Aid Deluxe Automatic BP3AR1-4DRITE

Any of these monitors would be a good choice and will cost you somewhere between sixty and eighty dollars. And each will automatically inflate the pressure cuff—pumping up a rubber bulb is not required. Just be sure the cuff fits your arm as we discussed earlier, and you're on your way. If you have hypertension and are on medication, you need one of these. And if you're borderline, I recommend having one as well. As far as where to find them, most can be purchased online.

So again, home monitoring is more accurate than office-based blood pressure measurements. That might come as a surprise, but that's what the best evidence tells us. So is this the best way to follow your BP? Nope. We'll answer that question next.

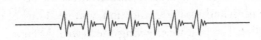

12

Ambulatory Blood Pressure Monitoring: The New Gold Standard

Being the gold standard of anything is a tall order, and especially when it comes to measuring blood pressure and diagnosing and managing hypertension. But ambulatory blood pressure monitoring (ABPM) lives up to its newfound reputation. First, we need to describe this technique.

ABPM involves wearing a device that takes blood pressure measurements over a twenty-four or forty-eight-hour period. It's not bulky or uncomfortable, and most people tolerate it without too many complaints. The monitor will measure your BP every fifteen to twenty minutes while you're awake and every thirty to sixty minutes while asleep. Data from ABPM is plugged into a computer and a twenty-four-hour average BP is determined. It may be possible to get usable info wearing it for as little as six to eight hours, but the longer the better.

Most devices can provide other data, but what we're really interested in is what our blood pressure is doing over an extended period of time. The information obtained is extremely accurate, and an average pressure greater than 130/80 will define the presence of hypertension. These numbers may seem a little low, but remember, this is an *average* blood pressure, and this threshold indicates probable excursions of your BP into a higher, more dangerous range.

How does this technique compare to office-based measurements? It's not called the gold standard for nothing. ABPM is much more accurate than the readings obtained at your doctor's office. And it's better than those measured at home, though home monitoring is closer to ABPM than are those taken at the office. So this establishes the pecking order of our methods of measuring blood pressure. The best is ABPM, followed by home monitoring, with those measurements in your doctor's office trailing the field.

The superiority of ABPM has been so well established that the British, in their National Institute for Health and Care Excellence (NICE) guidelines, state that if a person's blood pressure is elevated in the office, ambulatory BP measurements should be used to confirm the diagnosis of hypertension. If that person is unable or unwilling to tolerate ABPM, home monitoring should be done to establish the diagnosis. The guideline goes on to state that if an office blood pressure is elevated and ABPM is normal, the diagnosis should be white-coat syndrome rather than hypertension.

Experts in the US give largely the same recommendation as the Brits. ABPM should be used to establish the accurate diagnosis of hypertension and before the start of any medications. Once the diagnosis is made and treatment has begun, home monitoring should be encouraged, with measurements in the doctor's office used for confirmation only. Should these office BPs become too high or too low, another ABPM might be indicated with a treatment plan adjusted accordingly.

The bottom line here is that we should be doing more ambulatory blood pressure monitoring. But even though ABPM is the new gold standard, every silver lining has a cloud. This cloud is big and dark, and as is too often the case, has to do with money. The cost of ambulatory blood pressure monitoring varies somewhere between $100 and $350, depending on where you live and who's doing the testing.

This represents another instance where clinical experience, substantiated guidelines, and good medical care collide with those who are paying for it: our government and insurance companies. When managed properly, we know that the control of hypertension has the potential to significantly improve lives and ultimately save many dollars, and ABPM can clearly help do that. While they agree that ABPM is a worthwhile weapon in the fight against a powerful and unforgiving foe, our payers have until recently been unwilling to financially cover this service. Even today, they don't routinely pay for the total cost.

We can only hope that something will give here and that our gold standard will become affordable, accessible, and routinely incorporated into our practices. In the meantime, you'll need to ask your healthcare provider if they offer this monitoring, and if not, where you might be able to have it done.

By now, it should have become an important tool that we routinely use in our diagnosis and management of blood pressure problems. Until that day comes, stay away from drugstore and grocery store BP machines, work with your doctor's office to get the most accurate readings possible, and invest in a recommended home monitor.

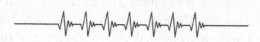

13

The White-Coat Syndrome

Is white-coat syndrome for real or just another old wives' tale perpetuated by wishful patients and their naïve healthcare providers? Let's see if we can figure it out.

Most experts agree this is an actual clinical condition, but how would they go about defining this problem? White-coat hypertension or white-coat syndrome is a condition in which some people have an elevated blood pressure in the doctor's office (or other clinical setting) but nowhere else. Home monitoring is usually normal, as well as readings taken at the drugstore or other nonthreatening location. Even though the cause is suspected to be increased anxiety while in the office, most of these individuals won't exhibit any evidence of a rapid heartbeat, flushing, or increased respirations—all signs of anxiety. That makes it difficult for us to determine who might be at risk for this, who really has high blood pressure and needs medication, and who doesn't.

In my experience, a lot of people come into the office and declare to the nurse wrapping a BP cuff around their arm, "I know my blood pressure's going to be high. I have white-coat syndrome." What should we do with that?

First, here are a couple of important caveats:

- While it's critical to have an accurate blood pressure reading, many offices and clinics use a cuff that is too small, making the measurement falsely high.

- A single reading should never be used to diagnose a person as having a normal blood pressure or of being hypertensive.

- Using an automated BP device, repeated over fifteen to twenty minutes, gives a more accurate measurement than a manual reading. These are becoming much more frequently utilized in medical offices, though waiting twenty minutes for repeated readings is impractical for most practices.

- Talking and fidgeting during BP measurement can cause an inaccurate reading.

- If you think you have the syndrome and have a blood pressure cuff at home, bring a log of your measurements and show this to your physician. That's always helpful.

So the first thing to do is be sure that the measurement in the office is as accurate as possible. Once we have that, and it's above normal, a couple of things need to happen. If you're convinced you have white-coat syndrome, your physician should recommend either home measurements with adequate equipment or ambulatory blood pressure monitoring (ABPM). We considered the importance of ABPM in the last chapter, but where white-coat syndrome is a factor, it is very useful if not essential. This gives us the most accurate information about what an individual's blood pressure is doing during an average day, with its normal fluctuations of stress and physical activity.

There's a bothersome flipside here, and it's called "masked hypertension." This occurs when a person's BP readings are normal in the office yet clearly elevated at a sustained level while being measured with an ABPM. That's really scary, but it happens. A one-time reading in the clinic might be normal or just a little high, while the rest of the day and night the BP is dangerously elevated. This is another reason why accurate blood pressure measurement is so important, and why I'm always happy to look at my patients' home readings.

Once white-coat syndrome has been diagnosed—elevated blood pressure in the office, normal BP measurements at home and by ABPM—what next? Can we just say, "Yeah, you've got the syndrome, so don't worry about it. Everything's fine."

Not so fast. As with anybody with an elevated blood pressure—

white-coat or sustained—we will need to check for any evidence of target organ damage. Remember, these are the areas where the constant hammering of hypertension causes problems—the brain, heart, and kidneys. If we find any evidence of these, that individual will need to have his blood pressure aggressively managed, probably with medication.

If there's no such evidence, we can take a more relaxed approach and follow that person routinely. However, we have to keep in mind that this is not necessarily a benign condition. Many people with the syndrome will go on to develop full-blown hypertension. Worse yet, before that becomes obvious, some will develop heart, brain, and kidney problems. We'll need to keep an eye on their blood pressure measured at home and monitor for any subsequent evidence of target organ damage.

The bottom line here? Yes, the white-coat syndrome is for real. It's not necessarily a benign condition and should raise a couple of red flags for those who have it. This is another instance where diet, exercise, weight management, smoking cessation—the things we should all be doing—are really important.

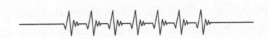

14

You Gotta Know Your Numbers

It's Getting a Little Frosty

"Now *this* is an interesting case."

Tim Brewster, a fourth-year medical student rotating through the ER, stopped beside me at the nurses' station and plopped the chart of room 4 on the counter.

"The guy can't stop itching," Tim said. "I mean, he's just clawing at himself."

I didn't look up, having my own conundrum in the ENT room to unravel. The patient was four years old and had a bead in his right ear and a piece of crayon in his nose. I wasn't sure where to start.

"I might need you to help me with this one, Dr. Lesslie," Tim added, sliding the medical record close to me. "He's miserable, and I'm not sure what to do."

I glanced at the chart and the chief complaint—*itching*. That seemed appropriate for our medical student to take a crack at. The patient was fifty-five years old, a male, and the complaint seemed simple enough.

"Utah Jones," I mused, noticing the man's name. "Interesting."

"I asked him about that," Tim said. "He told me his father was in the military and they traveled around a lot. Apparently he was born somewhere in Utah and that's how he got his name. Didn't stay out west for very long, though. I think he's lived in this area for most of his life."

"Tell me more about your patient, Tim. What do you think's going on?"

Tim straightened and took a deep breath. "Well, it's February, so the possibility of poison ivy or poison oak is pretty small, and—"

"Hold it just a second. What makes you say that?"

"It's winter, and all the leaves are gone, so I…you wouldn't expect…"

"Here's something interesting to keep in mind," I began, leaning an elbow on the countertop. "If someone is sensitive to poison ivy, they can get it by coming into contact with the roots of the plant or the stem—even in the middle of winter. It doesn't have to be the leaves. In fact, some of the worst cases I've seen have been in the dead of winter when someone was burning debris in their yard—limbs and leaves and stuff. Without knowing it, they were burning poison ivy, and the smoke caused a terrible reaction, including their eyes and mouth and upper airway."

Tim's eyes widened and he shook his head. "He didn't say anything about burning stuff, but I didn't ask…"

"That's okay. We'll find that out. Anything else here? Medications? Any unusual changes in his diet?"

"No, he doesn't take any prescription medicine. He told me he hadn't been to a doctor in more than twenty years, and wouldn't be here this afternoon if it wasn't for the itching."

My finger traced the "Allergies" box on the chart. Nothing. And nothing was listed under "Current Medications." I scanned the rest of his chart. My finger stopped over Utah's blood pressure: 180/110.

"What do you think about this?"

Tim's eyes focused on the numbers beneath my fingertip. "I guess I didn't notice that. He was scratching and clawing and asking for help. I just didn't…that's pretty high, isn't it?"

"Pretty high." I picked up the man's chart and headed around the nurses' station. "Come on, let's go talk with Utah."

Tim was right. Utah Jones sat on the stretcher of room 4 and clawed at his arms and legs and neck. He was miserable.

"I hope you can help me, Doc." He looked at me and his weathered face managed a smile. "I need some relief."

We talked for a few minutes and he never stopped scratching. My own skin was beginning to prickle and I fought the urge to rub my arms and legs.

Utah Jones had no history of any medical problems, and he again admitted his twenty-plus years with no medical attention.

I asked about any history of high blood pressure, and he shrugged. "I think someone might have mentioned that in the past, but that would be years ago. I think it was a GP somewhere, and he told me to cut down on my salt. Never been on any medicine for it though."

I examined his eyes and listened to his heart and lungs. But the diagnosis had been made when I had first pulled the curtain aside and walked into the room.

"We're going to get you something right now for your itching, Utah, and check a few things while you're here. We're going to need to get your blood pressure under control."

"Sure, Doc, as long as you can help me with this infernal itching."

At the nurses' station, I turned to Tim. "What do you want to do now?"

The medical student shuffled his feet and studied the ceiling tiles. "I guess some Benadryl? Maybe a shot to get things started?"

"How about a chest X-ray, EKG, and some lab work. And maybe a urinalysis?"

"Lab work? And an EKG? Why would we need that?"

"Did you notice his skin?" I started writing some orders on Utah's chart.

"His skin? You mean the dry patches? That's eczema, isn't it? I just thought with the dry air outside and the fact that he has sensitive skin…I thought it was eczema, but not too bad a case. It was just a little dry skin, and I don't think that would be causing his itching."

I nodded and continued making some notes on Utah's chart. "Ever heard of uremic frost?"

"Uremic what?"

"Uremic frost. It's a coating of crystalized urea—one of the main waste products we produce every day. Normally our kidneys take care of it, but when they're not functioning properly, the urea levels in our blood can increase to the point where it's excreted onto our skin. It crystalizes and forms that whitish film you see—the uremic frost. And it can cause irritation—and itching."

"Uremic. You mean kidney failure." Tim stared blankly. "His blood pressure. It's probably been high for a long time and now…"

"And now his kidneys are failing."

Utah's EKG showed evidence of a long history of strain—his heart had been working too hard and too long against a high blood pressure. His urinalysis showed a lot of protein and blood, evidence of poorly functioning kidneys. And his blood work confirmed the diagnosis of renal failure, with a sky-high creatinine level—another waste product our kidneys clear from our systems.

Tim stood behind me, peering over my shoulder at the lab reports. "Wow, that's pretty bad. But how are we going to help his itching? He didn't respond very much to the Benadryl."

I shook my head. "It's going to take more than that, I'm afraid."

The unit secretary answered her phone and looked up at me.

"They're ready for Mr. Jones in dialysis."

15

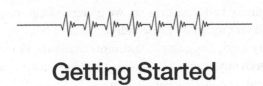

Getting Started

One of the things that makes the practice of medicine challenging, and at the same time very rewarding, is that we are all different. We don't all look the same or weigh the same. Some of us are tall and some are short. And then there's the whole issue of our genes. There's no question that some are blessed with good genes. It seems that no matter what they do, they're going to live to be a hundred. And then the rest of us, well, we seem to be genetically challenged with family histories loaded with diabetes, heart disease, and cancer.

Then there's personal preferences—where we live, how we spend our leisure time, how much we consider our health, and especially what we like to eat. That may be the most confounding factor. It appears there are even some of us who don't particularly like grits. Go figure.

So it's this uniqueness, this variability that teaches us that one size doesn't fit all. Those of us dedicated to improving the health and lives of our patients learn this reality early on in our careers. There's no cookie-cutter approach when it comes to dealing with complex medical problems such as hypertension, or many of the simple ones either. There's no magic bullet, no lightning in a bottle, no cure-all wonder drug. That's the reality, and the challenge.

So, how do we get started when it comes to managing problems with our blood pressure? The one place we all have in common, the one starting point that has to happen for each of us, is a tough, objective examination of our lifestyle. This is presented in the broadest use of the term, since from a medical standpoint, our lifestyle encompasses multiple facets of our lives. We're going to take a quick survey of some of these now, and a more in-depth look later. These are the things we do that impact our lives—some positive, some negative—and the things we *don't* do that might help us.

The first area we need to focus on is our *diet*—what we put into our bodies. We *are* in fact what we eat. That can sometimes be pretty scary. One of the amazing things about our body is its ability to make do with what we feed it. There is a certain amount of leeway when it comes to extracting the correct balance of proteins, carbohydrates, and fats from our GI tract. Our diets don't have to be perfect—few are—to give us what we need. But there is a limit.

Next we'll consider *exercise*—the simple act of keeping our bodies in motion. We'll consider why this is essential, what kinds of exercise are the most efficient, and what dangers lie in store for those of us who neglect this important part of our well-being. There's good news here as well. Mounting evidence clearly demonstrates we don't have to run marathons or compete in triathlons to have a big and positive impact on our health. Simple and painless activities are all that's required, and no matter what your age or physical condition, there's something for everyone.

One of the benefits of regular and adequate exercise is the reduction of *stress*. This is another important element of our unique lifestyle. Each of us lives with our own level of tension, and though some of us think we're immune to its negative effects, we are all subject to its wear and tear. But does stress really have something to do with our blood pressure? You bet-cha, and we'll see how and why that happens. But it's not hard to imagine, is it? We live in an anxious, stressed-out culture. Just look around. People rushing here and there—deadlines to meet, meetings to attend, projects to complete. And all before 9:00 a.m.

But all of this stress takes a toll on our health. Anxiety is clearly associated with the development of hypertension, heart disease, diabetes, and other significant problems. We need to identity the stressors in our lives and eliminate them, when possible. Again, it all turns out to be about balance. A little stress is healthy for us. It's when it overpowers us that things start breaking down.

One of the things that can break down is our *sleep*. This is another critical part of our well-being and it hinges on a healthy lifestyle. Inadequate sleep is a factor in the development of a lot of serious complications, including heart disease as well as diabetes and high blood pressure. We're going to explore simple ways to improve our sleep patterns, learn when it's important to undergo professional testing, and consider effective treatments when we have a real problem.

Sleep and high blood pressure? Yep, that's right. It all ties together—intricately interwoven. One aspect of our health impacts another and another and another. It's all about balance.

Our lifestyles embrace much more than we've briefly talked about so far, including our close and significant relationships, our spiritual health, even our dreams and aspirations. But we've got plenty to work with here, and we probably have changes we need to make. And even though Dave Jernigan wants to reach for that magic pill to lower his blood pressure, this is where we're going to start—examining our lifestyle. So let's get going.

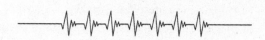

16

Don't DASH Off:
Your Diet as a Weapon Against
High Blood Pressure

When it comes to our health, diet—what we put into our bodies—is critically important. Some would rightly argue it's the cornerstone of an overall healthy lifestyle. Exercise, adequate sleep, less stress, no smoking—those are all significant factors in determining our physical health. But what we put into our mouths can quickly undo a lot of the good we might otherwise be achieving.

This is especially true when it comes to managing our blood pressure. Fortunately, there's a lot of good evidence to help us here. First, it should come as no surprise that it becomes easier to reach our blood pressure goal when we approach our ideal weight. This is based on our body mass index (BMI) number, something each of us should know. This is derived from a simple formula, and all you need to know is your height and weight. It's easy to find a table online to see where you are, and what you need to be doing. The bottom line though is that the more lean we are and the closer to our ideal BMI range we come, the easier it is to have a more normal blood pressure. That's not always a simple task—sometimes requiring significant lifestyle adjustments.

When it comes to making our diets our friends in our battle with hypertension, there are a couple of good options. The most familiar and most researched is something called the DASH diet. The **D**ietary **A**pproaches to **S**top **H**ypertension diet was developed by the National

Institutes of Health (NIH), a division of the Department of Health and Human Services, in an effort to help control and even prevent high blood pressure. This guideline has been around for almost twenty-five years and has been proven time and again to be effective, safe, and easily incorporated into our varied and busy lifestyles. But what is it?

Well, it's not magic. This diet stresses an increased consumption of vegetables, fruits, whole grains, nuts, beans, lean meats (as well as fish and poultry), and low-fat dairy products. It also recommends a significant reduction in sugar, red meat, and added fats. One of its goals is to increase the amounts of calcium, magnesium, and potassium in our diets, all of which are important for a variety of reasons, including healthy blood vessels and lower blood pressure. Up to this point, it might sound a lot like the Mediterranean Diet, and it should, since they are very similar. We'll talk about that dietary approach a little later.

But what sets the DASH diet apart from other diets is its emphasis on reducing the amount of salt we consume daily. We Americans consume on average more than 3500 mgs of salt a day—somewhere around two teaspoons. Some of us may be thinking, *Wow, I have that much before lunchtime.* It's easy to reach that level when you consider the saltshaker on the table, our salt-loaded processed foods, and the salt content of your favorite fast foods or snacks. We also know this level of salt intake is dangerous, and a major contributor to the development of high blood pressure. The DASH diet recommends lowering this intake to less than 2300 mgs a day—a number endorsed by the American Heart Association. There's even a "lower sodium" DASH diet that puts the number at 1500 mgs. It turns out that's where we're going to need to be, but this goal takes some work and palate adjustment.

Is it worth it? Does the DASH diet really make a difference? Well, here's what we know. After as little as four to six weeks on the diet, individuals with hypertension can reduce their systolic pressure by as much as 11 millimeters of mercury (mm Hg), and their diastolic by 6. If a new blood pressure medicine achieved these kinds of results in a research trial, the authors (and drug manufacturer) would be ecstatic. This is the equivalent of what we hope to accomplish with the use of a single BP medication. So yes, this dietary approach makes a difference. The good news for those of us with borderline or even normal pressures, this diet can lower those numbers by 6 mm Hg and 3 mm Hg—again, an important reduction.

So it works. And not only does it help with hypertension, there's also good evidence that it can help prevent heart disease, diabetes, certain cancers, and osteoporosis. But what does it look like?

The Mayo Clinic has some very helpful information (found at www .mayoclinic.org/health-lifestyle/nutrition-and-healthy-eating/in-depth/ dash-diet/art-20050989) about this diet. Basically, it recommends four to five servings of vegetables each day, six to eight servings of grain, four to five of fruits, two to three of dairy, six or fewer of lean meats, poultry, and fish, and two to three of fats and oils. It limits the servings of nuts, seeds, and legumes to four to five a *week*, and sweets to less than five, also per week. It needs to be stressed that the DASH diet is not intended to be a weight-reduction guideline. This was designed to address hypertension and it does that effectively.

We mentioned the Mediterranean Diet and its similarities to the DASH diet. This is a good example of where we need to experiment a little—maybe even mix and match. There are really important elements in the DASH diet—lowering salt intake, increasing calcium and potassium and magnesium—but it's not going to help you lose weight. The Mediterranean Diet is more effective with this, since it puts more limits on your carbohydrates while stressing nuts, legumes, and olive oil. This diet makes a lot of sense to me, and we've tried to incorporate it into our own lifestyles, while at the same time trying to significantly limit our salt intake. There are numerous websites for this, but a concise outline can be found at www.nlm.nih.gov/medlineplus/ency/patientinstructions/000110.htm.

So now you know about the DASH diet, and that there are several ways that what we eat can help (or hurt) us in our effort to control our blood pressures. It's not rocket science, it's within everyone's reach, and it can be done. That's the good news.

17

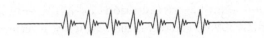

The Low-Carb Approach

We've looked at the DASH diet and how it's well suited to help you lower your blood pressure. But one size doesn't fit all, and each of us might need to experiment a little to find our ideal diet—one we can live with.

However, I'm convinced that whatever diet we choose, it needs to limit our carbohydrate intake. But what's so bad about carbs? Why the rap against our comfort foods? Let's start with the real culprit here—*insulin*. This is something we really need to understand.

Our body needs energy to grow and survive. We get that from three sources: carbohydrates, proteins, and fats. We are able to derive energy from each of these classes of nutrients, but carbs are the easiest, quickest source—and in the long run, the most harmful. That's because in order to utilize the energy in carbs, we must have the action of the hormone insulin.

Insulin is made in the beta cells of the pancreas, and it's a relatively simple chain of fifty-one amino acids. Its release is signaled by the presence of carbohydrates in our bloodstream. When this process is initiated, insulin circulates throughout the body, seeking and attaching itself to insulin receptors. These are chemical binders located on the membranes of target cells, and once the insulin molecule combines with this receptor, the hormone is able to exert its actions, which are many.

Insulin directly or indirectly affects almost every tissue in our body. These actions are complex and interwoven, but right now, we're mainly considering how it interacts with glucose and how it affects the production of energy. It does this by its action on three tissues: the liver, muscles, and adipose tissue (fat).

Glucose—the simplest and most basic sugar—can be immediately used for energy throughout the body, or it can be stored in the liver as glycogen. Once stored, this complex of modified glucose molecules can be readily and rapidly used as an energy source when needed. Excess glucose can be converted into fat and stored in our adipose tissue. Getting the energy out of this fat is a more complex process than burning available glucose and it takes a little longer. That's why our bodies first burn and deplete the available glucose and then our glycogen stores before finally turning to our adipose tissue. And that's one of the reasons it's so hard to get rid of unwanted fat.

Every carbohydrate we put into our body eventually becomes glucose—some quicker than others. But even the highly touted complex carbohydrates end up as circulating glucose. All carbs, from simple to complex, end up as glucose and all activate the release of insulin.

The first thing this hormone does is move glucose into the cells of various tissues. As we noted earlier, this is done by attaching itself to the cell's insulin receptor. You may have heard of or even been told that you have some degree of "insulin resistance." A cell's insulin receptor is the location where that resistance takes place. The receptors seem to wear down over time after repeatedly being called into action due to a persistently high-carb diet. More and more insulin is required to activate the signal and allow glucose to enter the cell.

You see where this leads—more and more insulin required to do the same amount of work and handle the same sugar load. The beta cells of the pancreas finally say, "I'm getting too old for this," and stop working. And that condition? Right—adult-onset diabetes. If this theory is correct, we should have an epidemic of diabetes on our hands given our colossal consumption of carbohydrates. And guess what. We do.

But back to the actions of insulin. It drives glucose into the cells of the liver, where it stimulates the formation of glycogen. It drives glucose into muscle cells, where it can be immediately burned for energy. And it drives glucose into the cells of our adipose tissue, where it promotes the storage of triglycerides in our fat cells.

Insulin has been called "the hormone of plenty." When we have plenty to eat, and a lot of glucose circulating throughout our bodies, insulin rapidly converts some of this to needed energy. The rest is stored away for a rainy day in the form of glycogen or as fat.

The problem with this rainy day business is that, in this country, that day never comes. Three not-so-square meals a day is the norm, with a few snacks thrown in for good measure. But our pancreas doesn't know that, and each time we load ourselves with carbs, insulin does what it's supposed to do: burn sugar and store fat—taking advantage of this moment of plenty and preparing for more austere, less plentiful times.

Along the way, it can elevate our blood pressures, which is what we're really concerned about here. It can also damage the walls of our arteries and interfere with the normal clotting that takes place in these vessels, leading to the formation of atherosclerotic plaques. There is even emerging evidence that excess levels of insulin may be associated with the development of several cancers, including those of the colon, ovary, and breast.

Lest I give you a completely one-sided view of this essential hormone, insulin does some important and beneficial things. It does handle glucose for us, and it is important in the growth process and the formation of proteins. The problem is that it was never intended to handle the kinds of carbohydrate loads we throw at our pancreas.

The bottom line: we all need to reduce the amount of carbohydrates we consume. It doesn't matter whether we're talking about whole grains, complex carbs, or multigrain whatever. We need to know the carb content of what we're putting into our bodies and lower it.

That brings up a frequent and important question: What constitutes a low-carb diet? How many daily grams of carbs is okay?

Some general but useful guidelines are available here. Robert Atkins (of the Atkins Diet fame) would tell us that the cutoff should be 30 to 45 grams per day. That's hard, considering that one piece of whole-wheat bread has 23 grams, and one medium banana contains 26 grams.

A more realistic approach would be to target 60 or so grams per day, knowing that it's impossible to identify and eliminate every single carb from your diet. And we don't want to, anyway. A certain amount of carbs is essential for our well-being. We just need to find a way to limit their intake and restore the balanced diet our systems were designed to handle. It won't take something as drastic as the Atkins Diet, though that might be a good place to start for a couple of weeks. Fortunately, we have some effective alternatives, diets that will get the job done and that we can live with long-term.

We'll take a look at some of these next.

(For a great discussion of our hunter-gatherer origins, I recommend the book *Protein Power* by Michael R. Eades and Mary Dan Eades. And for a complete discussion of the importance of low-carb diets, two books you should look at are *60 Ways to Lower Your Blood Sugar* by Dennis Pollock and *The New Sugar Busters!* by H. Leighton Steward and others. These are all great resources and will help clarify the mistakes and myths of the past few decades regarding what we should and should not be eating.)

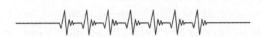

18

Please Pass the Salt
(No, Please *Pass* on the Salt)

"Robert, if you keep putting so much salt on your food, there will come a day when you won't be able to use any. You'll have high blood pressure and heart trouble."

Thus spoke my paternal grandmother, Bobo. The words struck fear into the heart of this six-year-old boy, and I never forgot them, to this day casting guarded glances at every saltshaker that crosses my path.

Bobo was right, of course. We all know that salt is not our friend, though we remain addicted to its briny allure. French fries with no salt? Salt-less popcorn? Homemade pasta sauce with no…You get the picture. Salt in our food is everywhere, and that's the way we like it. But at the same time, we probably are all aware of its central and complicating role in high blood pressure. How does this pristine, simple compound cause such sinister and stealthy damage to our bodies? Before we look into that, let's consider the history of this naturally occurring and fascinating mineral.

Salt has been an important part of the human story for thousands of years. Much more than a seasoning for our food, it has served critical functions extending from our distant past into our modern times. Perhaps the most significant of these was its use in the preservation of food. This allowed for more extended travel over uncharted areas of the globe, as well as providing for survival during times of famine, prolonged winters, and unforeseen causes of crop failure.

While our grocery store shelves are stacked with an inexpensive abundance of these white crystals, such has not always been the case. In fact, the production of salt—either through mining or the evaporation of sea water—was costly and time-consuming. If a large and easily accessible deposit of salt was located, a town or city quickly sprang up nearby. Such deposits have been found in New York, Texas, Ohio, Kansas, Nova Scotia, and Ontario, and in several familiar places in Europe, such as Salzburg, Austria, which means "the city of salt."

The presence of this commodity allowed large and affluent cities and city-states to quickly develop and become major trading centers. However, with affluence comes greed and covetousness—a time-honored and proven recipe for hostile activity and war. Such was the case with many of these salt centers, and numerous military campaigns were waged in the procurement of this important compound.

The importance of salt was not lost upon some of the writers of the Old Testament. Moses (in Leviticus 2:13) and the writer of Ezra (Ezra 7:21-22) are two examples that demonstrate the high regard in which this mineral was held.

More importantly, Jesus, in Matthew 5:13, uses salt as an important metaphor—one that still informs us. As His followers, we are instructed to be "the salt of the earth." Not only are we to add flavor to the world around us—through service, love, and caring—but we are called to preserve the communities around us, to protect the helpless, and to live the gospel. With this admonition comes the warning that if the salt loses its flavor, "it is no longer good for anything, except to be thrown out and trampled underfoot." A lot to think about.

Fortunately, we're no longer dealing with wars being fought over salt, or with the salting of farmland. Our battles with this mineral are much more subtle—unseen and silent, but no less devastating.

Bobo's words still ring in my ears. While she might not have known the important history of salt, nor the nuances of its effects on our blood vessels and heart, she was on to something. And she was right.

But just *how* do these innocuous, white crystals cause us so much damage? This is important stuff, and critical to our understanding and management of high blood pressure. Let's take a look.

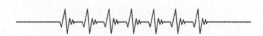

19

Wreaking Havoc: The Hidden Dangers in Your Saltshaker

"And don't forget to cut down your salt intake."

If you have hypertension, you've probably been told that dozens of times, maybe more. It's a part of every path to a lower blood pressure and apparently we need to be reminded of it frequently. But what does "cutting down" mean? And why is it important? Let's start with the *important* part.

The connection between sodium intake and the development of high blood pressure has been clearly established. For example, we know that primary hypertension (the kind that's not associated with a specific underlying cause) mainly occurs in areas of the world where dietary sodium exceeds 2.3 grams a day. It turns out to be rare where that intake is less than 1.2 grams. Less sodium, less hypertension.

It's important here to define some terms and make sure we refer to the same things. Salt is the compound containing sodium and chloride. If you noticed, the above numbers refer to *sodium*, not salt, and 2.3 grams of sodium would be the equivalent of about 6 grams of salt. In other words, 6 grams of salt (5.69 grams is the equivalent of 1 teaspoon of salt) contains 2.3 grams of sodium. This becomes important when we read dietary labels and consider specific recommendations.

So, 6 grams a day of *salt* appears to be the threshold where bad things start to happen. We need to keep that number in mind, and the fact that this is only *1 teaspoon!* Think about that for a moment. A single teaspoon a day is where things head south, and it turns out to be the maximum amount recommended by most experts. We'll talk about that later, but let's return to the relationship between sodium and high blood pressure.

Where salt intake is higher, the incidence of hypertension is higher. As further proof of this association, we know that when dietary salt is restricted, blood pressure falls, independent of any other intervention. That's important, and that's why we constantly hear "cut down on your salt."

But how and why does salt make your blood pressure go up? We know a lot about this, but not everything. For instance, we are aware of something called *sodium sensitivity.* Individuals respond differently to dietary sodium, with some being more sensitive than others. Their blood pressures go up much higher than those not sensitive. Most of us are sensitive, but this varies. We know that sensitivity increases with age and that it is more marked in obese individuals, African-Americans, patients with chronic kidney disease, and those with the metabolic syndrome. (There it is again—the dreaded Syndrome X.)

So, with those of us who are sodium sensitive, its ingestion causes a "volume expansion" of our circulating blood/plasma due to the increase in dissolved electrolytes (sodium and chloride). As a protective reflex, our blood pressure rises, causing an increase in the blood passing through our kidneys—all this in an effort to rid ourselves of the excess sodium and restore what should be our normal blood volume. The problem is that while our kidneys work overtime trying to eliminate this salt, we are busy dumping more into the system. When it rains, it pours. After a while, our blood pressure just stays elevated, and our arteries begin to lose their ability to dilate, compounding the problem. It's a vicious cycle, and a deadly one.

Just how deadly? Consider these projections. If each of us in the United States was able to limit our salt intake to a little less than half a teaspoon each day, we would experience the following benefits:

- The development of new cases of coronary heart disease would decrease by as many as 120,000 a year.
- Deaths in this country from *any* cause would decline by up to 92,000 a year.

• Healthcare costs would be reduced by almost 25 billion
  dollars.

Another sobering statistic is that high salt intake (more than a teaspoon
a day) potentially causes as many as 1.7 million deaths a year throughout
the world. To put that in a little perspective, that's more than the deaths
due to respiratory infections (1.6 million), HIV (1.5 million), diabetes (1.5
million), and road injuries/MVAs (1.3 million).

Seems obvious that we should all want to cut back on the amount
of salt we consume, but it's not that easy. Reaching for that saltshaker is
ingrained in our psyches—a reflex that will be hard to overcome. Understanding the importance of doing this is the first step. The next is to
become a little smarter, a little more salt savvy. Let's see how we go about
doing that.

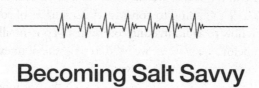

20

Becoming Salt Savvy

From the last chapter, we learned that more than one teaspoon of salt a day is associated with the development of high blood pressure and significant health problems. Because of that, most national and international health organizations (including the US Department of Agriculture and the Department of Health and Human Services) recommend daily consumption of less than that amount. They recommend a further reduction, as little as about a half teaspoon a day, if an individual falls into one or more of the following categories:

- age fifty-one years and older
- has an existing diagnosis of diabetes
- has an existing diagnosis of hypertension
- African-American
- has been diagnosed with chronic kidney disease

That represents a lot of us—in fact, most of us. We need to think about this teaspoon business a little more. That's not much. If you're a french-fry eater, just watch the cook behind the counter with their oversized shaker. That teaspoon threshold is reached pretty fast. This is where we need to be smart.

You might be thinking that most of our salt comes from the food we eat, and you'd be right—the saltshaker on the kitchen table, salt added while cooking, the salted snacks we all crave. Processed foods are notoriously high in salt content, as are many of the beverages we consume every day, such as your favorite cola. Some of these sources are obvious—salted or "brined" fish and meat, as well as most canned vegetables—while others are sneakier. We're going to consider these sources of sodium in our diets and learn how to avoid making common and potentially dangerous mistakes. But before we do that, we need to be aware of unexpected ways that salt can make its way into our lives.

Several common chemical ingredients used during food processing contain significant amounts of sodium. These should be listed on the food's label (usually in small print) and include mono*sodium* glutamate (MSG), *sodium* saccharin, *sodium* phosphates (used as stabilizers), *sodium* benzoate and nitrite (preservatives), and *sodium* citrate. Baking soda (sodium bicarbonate) is another source.

Commonly used over-the-counter medications, including many antacids, can contain bothersome amounts of sodium. Keep in mind the limit of *2,300 mgs* of sodium a day and consider the following:

Alka-Seltzer—521 mgs/dose
Mylanta-II—160 mgs/100ml
Bromo-Seltzer—717 mgs/dose
Metamucil—250 mgs/dose
Rolaids—53 mgs/dose
Di-Gel—170 mgs/100ml

It sneaks up on us and it all adds up. But there's more.

Our drinking water, depending on where we live, can have significant amounts of sodium. If you have a well and use a water softener, this is almost always some form of salt and will raise the sodium level. The harder the water, the more sodium needed to treat it. If you use well water, and especially if you have it treated, you should have it analyzed.

All of these can be significant sources of sodium, but let's return to our food, the most important source of our salt and the most readily identified and corrected. So let's see what we know or *think* we know. The Food and Drug Administration (FDA) provides us with some interesting information, including the "10 types of foods" that provide more than 40 percent of the sodium we ingest. Before reading on, give this some thought, and see which ones you can guess.

Soups
Breads and rolls
Snacks (chips, pretzels, popcorn, crackers)
Cold cuts and cured meats
Pizza
Processed poultry
Sandwiches (including hamburgers, hot dogs, and subs)
Cheese (both natural and processed)
Mixed pasta dishes (lasagna, spaghetti with meat sauce)
Mixed meat dishes (meat loaf, beef stew, chili)

These are pretty obvious, though you might have been surprised by a few.

Now let's consider some of the big offenders, and some of the things that are "sodium friendly." A few of these surprised me as well. (This data comes from the Texas A&M AgriLife Extension and can be found at http://fcs.tamu.edu/food_and_nutrition/pdf/sodium-content-of-your-food-b1400.pdf. This is a great site with a lot of useful information.) These are presented as one serving, with the associated sodium content.

Brewed coffee—2 mgs

Cocoa mix—232 mgs

Canned apple juice—16 mgs

Canned lemonade—60 mgs

Imported mineral water—42 mgs

Natural blue cheese—396 mgs

Regular and low-fat cottage cheese—457 mgs

Feta cheese—316 mgs

Parmesan, grated—528 mgs

Parmesan, hard—454 mgs

American cheese spread—381 mgs

Whipped cream—4 mgs

Whole milk—122 mgs

Whole low-sodium milk—6 mgs

Chocolate ice cream—75 mgs

Soft-serve vanilla ice milk—163 mgs

Ready-to-serve chocolate pudding—262 mgs

Yogurt with fruit—133 mgs

One egg—59 mgs

Black sea bass—57 mgs

Catfish (for us Southerners)—50 mgs

Smoked herring—5,234 mgs (good luck!)

Canned pink salmon—443 mgs

Canned tuna—288 mgs

Canned crab—425 mgs

Boiled lobster—212 mgs

Fried shrimp—225 mgs

Cooked bacon—274 mgs

Canadian bacon—394 mgs

Ham (3 oz)—1,114 mgs!

Cooked lean veal—69 mgs

Chicken frankfurter—617 mgs

Beef frankfurter—639 mgs

Kielbasa—280 mgs

Frozen meat loaf dinner—
 1,304 mgs!

One banana—2 mgs

One-half grapefruit—1 mg

Salted peanuts—986 mgs

The list goes on and on, with some pretty interesting info. And to make another point, consider this:

Raw asparagus (4 spears)—4 mgs
Frozen asparagus (4 spears)—4 mgs
Regular canned asparagus (4 spears)—298 mgs

This is an important point, and something we should all keep in mind. Canned, in a bag, through a fast-food window: eventually it's gonna get ya.

So what are we to do? Once again, the FDA provides us with some solid information (www.fda.gov/Food/ResourcesForYou/Consumers/ucm315393.htm). Here's my take on what they have to say:

1. Pay attention to the nutrition labels on your food and beverages. Check the sodium content, remembering your daily target of less than 2,300 mgs. When available, read the fine print, searching for those hidden sources of sodium we discussed earlier.

2. Avoid processed foods whenever possible. Prepare your own food when you can and limit the salt used in cooking. Try keeping the saltshaker off the table.

3. Add flavor to your food without adding salt. Experiment with herbs and spices, such as rosemary, oregano, basil, curry powder, garlic, and various peppers. If you choose a seasoning blend, check the sodium content. If you really like it, it's probably really loaded.

4. Buy fresh food when you can, not processed. Frozen vegetables usually contain very little sodium, so this is a good choice. Check out the salt content of processed meats

(luncheon meats, sausages, and corned beef) and choose fresh poultry, pork, and lean meat.

5. Watch your vegetables. Sure, we need to be eating more of these, but keep an eye out for the sodium content if you're not buying fresh or frozen. Remember, most canned vegetables are loaded with salt.

6. Rinse your food whenever possible. This is true in a general way for fruits and vegetables, but canned foods (tuna, vegetables, beans) can also be rinsed, removing some of the added sodium.

7. Examine your dairy products. Avoid processed cheese products and spreads. Instead, choose fat-free or low-fat milk and milk products (yogurt, cheese, and soy milk).

8. Switch to unsalted snacks. Remember the sodium content of dry roasted peanuts? A single serving is 968 mgs. Choose unsalted nuts and seeds, and avoid those chips and pretzels. It takes some getting used to, but you can avoid a lot of sodium and unneeded carbs and calories.

9. Think about your condiments. Ketchup, salad dressings, soy sauce, and many seasoning packets contain significant amounts of sodium. Try experimenting with no-salt-added ketchup, add oil and vinegar to your salad rather than salad dressing, and limit your amount of seasonings from flavoring packets.

10. When you're eating out, *watch* out! This turns out to be really important. I recently read that for the first time ever, Americans are spending more in restaurants (including fast-food) than in grocery stores. Think about that for a moment. This is probably a function of our increasingly busy lifestyles. We don't have time to buy groceries and prepare a meal. That's something we can all understand. But restaurants typically load their food with salt, so you have to be on your guard. Ask for your food to be prepared with no salt, or choose a lower-sodium option if available. And don't reach for that saltshaker. It'll raise your blood pressure and that of the chef.

These are all good points we need to keep in mind. Later, we'll look at *balance* in our lives, and how it applies to each and every facet, including our health. It also applies to watching our salt intake. We need to be aware of the dangers of too much sodium and work to reduce the amount we ingest. But we need to do it without becoming obsessed—constantly reading labels and measuring every grain. The good news is that it *can* be done and with balance. What we will find is that our craving for salt will gradually diminish and we can become salt free. Or nearly so. And that's going to help our blood pressures.

21

Exercise: Get Moving

You know what's coming next. We hear it all the time—"Get up and do something! Don't become a couch potato."

We know we should be exercising, but sometimes it's hard to get started. Where do we find the motivation for that first step or first push-up? Maybe we need to start with the *why* and then figure out the *how*.

It turns out the *why* is pretty overwhelming. The list of the benefits of physical activity is long and sometimes surprising.

As we would expect, exercise has a positive (protective) effect on the development of many common chronic conditions—heart disease, diabetes, chronic lung disease, kidney disease, and some kinds of cancers. Some experts believe the risk of recurrent breast cancer can be lowered by as much as 50 percent and the risk of developing colon cancer by up to 60 percent. Alzheimer's disease falls into this category as well—something that should get the attention of those of us in our middle-years and beyond. And it should come as no surprise that physical activity reduces the incidence of obesity, with all the problems associated with being overweight.

Now here are a few surprising benefits. The risk of osteoporosis is reduced with weight-bearing exercise. There is actually an increase in bone mineral density, with a demonstrated reduction in the possibility of suffering a hip or other type of fracture. And since physical activity improves muscle tone and balance, the chances of falling are significantly diminished. We also see a decrease in the incidence and severity of arthritis.

Exercise also reduces risk of gallstones as well as improving brain functioning. Regular physical activity can reduce stress and help lessen anxiety and depression. We previously mentioned that vigorous exercise can help you get to sleep faster and that it can be deeper and more efficient.

When it comes to blood pressure, the benefits are important and straightforward. We know that regular exercise can significantly lower our systolic and diastolic pressures—by as much as 5 to 15 mm Hg. Those are big numbers, especially considering that each 5 mm Hg reduction in systolic blood pressure can reduce our risk of stroke by almost 15 percent. And exercise can improve the health of our blood vessels.

With most of these benefits, this appears to be "dose-related"—the longer and more vigorous the exercise, the greater the improvements we experience. But how much is enough, and what kinds of exercise are we talking about?

Let's first think about the *what*. We'll consider the two main types of exercise: aerobic and resistance training. Aerobic exercises include brisk walking, running, bike riding, and the various machines that taunt us at the gym: treadmills, elliptical trainers, stair-steppers. This type of exercise has the greatest effect on our blood pressure and vessels, and is something each of us needs to be doing. If we are unable to walk or jog, swimming is a great alternative and will give us the same benefits without banging away at our knees, hips, and backs.

Resistance training—both weight lifting and isometric maneuvers— is also able to reduce our blood pressure. Seems peculiar to me, straining red-faced to lift a barbell off the floor. But it works, though not quite as effectively as aerobic activities. The main thing is to make exercising a natural and regular part of your life. Combining different types is a good idea, depending on your abilities, body type, and personal preferences.

Now the *how much*. Without getting too complicated, it might be helpful to consider how exercise physiologists measure exercise levels. They use the term MET (metabolic equivalents) to compare various forms of physical activity. For instance, 1 MET equals the amount of oxygen an adult would consume while sitting at rest for one minute. *Moderate* physical activity (swimming, general housecleaning, using a push mower, leisurely biking, and walking briskly at 3 to 5 miles per hour) would fall in the 3 to 6 METS range. *Vigorous* activity would be those things performed at greater than 6 METS and include running, push-ups and pull-ups, and jumping rope. (Try *that* sometime if you really want a good workout.

So with those definitions in mind, what should be our goals? Here are a few suggestions and examples:

- Vigorous exercise of at least 20 minutes three times a week, combined with 30 minutes of moderate activity on most days, has been associated with a 50 percent reduced risk of death in men and women aged fifty to seventy-one years.

- Another option is to combine 150 minutes of moderate exercise with 75 minutes of vigorous exercise each week.

And for those of us who fall in the category of "overly compulsive," we can use METS to quantify our activity level. Solid experimental evidence indicates that an expenditure of 500 to 1000 METS a week is necessary to achieve "substantial health benefits" (which interestingly these researchers define as a significant reduction in the risk of premature death and breast cancer). This equates to 150 minutes of walking each week (at 3.3 METS per minute, that gives you about 500). If so inclined, you can do the rest of the math to reach 1000, combining various physical activities.

Measuring your heart rate, while sometimes helpful, is *not* necessary, thus saving us money on various monitors and contraptions. As we can see, the key factors are *time* and *intensity.*

"But Dr. Lesslie," someone might say, "I *am* a couch potato. Shouldn't I have my doctor check me over before I start an exercise program?"

The answer is…maybe. But probably not. If you're in good health and don't have a history of a significant medical problem (heart disease, diabetes, uncontrolled high blood pressure), it's probably okay to get started. But start slowly and build from there.

On the other hand, if you fall into one of those categories, it will be a good idea to talk with your physician about how and when to begin. Be prepared though. If you ask ten doctors this question, you'll probably get eleven different answers.

If in doubt about the need for a medical evaluation before beginning a vigorous exercise program, there are a couple of questionnaires that will help guide you. You can find these at www.ncwc.edu/files/AHA.pdf.

The main point here is pretty simple—we need to get moving and keep moving. Oh, and it's never too late to start—as in *today.*

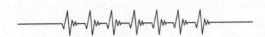

22

Hot Off the Press:
How Much Exercise to Live Longer?

We just looked at the importance of exercise in keeping our blood pressures under control, and at some of the other benefits we receive by being active. I just opened my mail and found a medical journal with an article that speaks directly to this issue of exercise and living longer. The authors, writing in the *Journal of the American College of Cardiology*, present information that is interesting and helpful. Here's the gist of what they had to say.

- It has been estimated that somewhere between 40 percent and 80 percent of the world's population is *sedentary*.

- Recent studies indicate that more than half of US adults do not follow current recommendations to engage in thirty minutes of moderate-intensity exercise per day, or seventy-five minutes of vigorous-intensity exercise per week.

- Current data indicates that only five to ten minutes per day of running or fifteen minutes per day of brisk walking can extend life expectancy by *three years*.

- Brief running (as little as five minutes per day) can reduce all-cause mortality by as much as 30 percent and deaths due to cardiovascular disease by up to 45 percent.

- This appears to be the "magic threshold": five minutes of running each day or fifteen minutes of brisk walking. Doing more than that can yield greater benefits, as we discussed in the last chapter, but can also precipitate overuse injuries.

- The flipside is that remaining sedentary or inactive can be associated with a 25 percent increased risk of developing heart disease and a 45 percent chance of dying from cardiovascular disease. Big numbers.

That's the short and sweet of it. Another compelling reason to get moving. We can live three years longer by walking briskly for only fifteen minutes a day. That ought to get our attention.

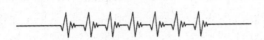

23

The Motor's Always Running: Chronic Stress and Your Blood Pressure

Frank Billings, a physician who practiced almost one hundred years ago, made the connection between high blood pressure and chronic stress. This is what he had to say about "nervous individuals":

> By the term *nervous* is meant a group of patients with nervous temperament who are high-strung, intense, always keyed up to a high pitch, always "on the go," never relaxing, whose motors always run at high speed. This group doesn't know how to play, but are Rooseveltian [Teddy, not FDR] in that they are intense in all they do, and a vacation means but a change in more strenuous work. These patients are always prompt in their appointments, are exacting, and in business very successful.

Sound familiar? Unfortunately, that description fits a lot of us. And Billings was right when he made the connection between his type A patients and hypertension. It makes sense that stress and anxiety—being keyed up to a high pitch—can elevate our blood pressures.

You know the feeling—flushed face, heartbeat pounding in your ears, sweaty palms, breath catching in your throat. It's another stress reaction—your body responding to some real or imagined threat.

This is a normal reaction, something our Creator has equipped us with, and it's usually helpful. The old fight-or-flight response has saved many of us through the centuries. We're swimming at the beach, glance behind us, and see the fin of a great white shark. Our brain responds in a split second. Adrenaline courses through our body, our heart rate speeds up, blood pressure rises, muscles tense, lungs work like mad, and our GI tracts shut down (hopefully). We also experience a temporary reduction in our hearing and develop tunnel vision, becoming locked in and focused on the threat in front of us. At the same time, cortisol, another stress hormone, floods our system, further raising our blood pressure and driving up our glucose level. We're ready—our energy level has boosted to warp speed, our muscles primed and waiting.

(This might not be the best example. We're not going to be able to successfully fight off this great white, and we're not going to outswim him either. But you get the picture.)

Anyway, this fight-or-flight response is something we regularly experience. While physical stressors and threats were the main factors activating this response in the past, our emotions now seem to be the prime culprits: anger, hate, fear, challenge, even love and joy. All of these are intense feelings and can trigger a stress response. It might not be a great white shark swimming nearby, but how about that boss storming down the hallway to your office? Or those blue flashing lights in the rearview mirror? Or your mother-in-law appearing in your driveway for an unexpected visit? Face flushes, heart rate speeds up…

It seems some of us, referred to as "hot reactors," are more affected than others. I know I'm one. The phone rings at 2:00 a.m., and I'm startled from a sound sleep. My heart pounds in my ears, my face flushes, and I start sweating. It appears a hot reactor can be identified at an early age. One large study looked at a group of teenagers and young adults, monitoring their vital signs while exposing them to various types of stress. One of these stressors was playing video games, and the researchers found a significant number of subjects experiencing elevations in their blood pressures while being glued to their screens. More worrisome was the finding that a majority of these individuals went on to develop full-fledged hypertension as they approached their twenties and thirties. So it starts early and might be something we can identify and modify. Hmm…maybe every Xbox should come with a blood pressure cuff.

So, we have this stress response, and fortunately it lasts only a few minutes and then gradually diminishes and disappears. No harm, no foul. The problem arises when this level of arousal becomes sustained—maybe not at the flushed-face level but just beneath that intensity. Our heart rate remains a little above normal, our blood pressure edges skyward, we have a sense that our face is hot—though not beet-red—and there is an overall feeling of being on edge. These symptoms wax and wane but may never completely go away.

This heightened stress—hovering just below the fight-or-flight mode—does a lot of damage to our bodies as well as to our spirits. We know that chronic stress is clearly connected to the development of diabetes, obesity, osteoporosis, and cardiovascular disease. In addition, we also know that this constant tension produces a heightened level of inflammatory markers in our bodies. This has been shown to be associated with an increased incidence of asthma, rheumatoid arthritis, and various forms of dermatitis. And we know that constant stress is linked to hypertension.

Just how does this happen, and how strong is the connection between chronic stress and our blood pressure? Let's go back for a moment to the fight-or-flight response. Remember, this is a natural response, finely tuned and usually beneficial. The chemicals and hormones released are designed to help us survive, and they are potent. We've mentioned the two main actors here: adrenaline and cortisol. Let's take another look at adrenaline.

This chemical is also known as epinephrine, and it's produced in our adrenal glands (hence its name *adrenal*-ine). We've already mentioned that it can affect our heart and cardiovascular system, causing an increase in heart rate and elevation in blood pressure. When this continues indefinitely, problems develop.

In my book *60 Ways to Lower Your Cholesterol*, I also discuss what a persistently elevated level of adrenaline can do to our lipids. We see an increase in triglyceride levels (free fatty acids) as well as elevated amounts of cholesterol. Adrenaline also causes a release of insulin, which further elevates our blood pressure and wreaks havoc with our normal lipid metabolism, while enhancing the formation of plaques in our arteries. None of this sounds very good, and it isn't.

The other powerful hormone associated with our stress response is *cortisol*. As with adrenaline, it's also produced in our adrenal glands. It does some important things and is essential in short bursts, raising our blood pressure and increasing the amount of available glucose in our blood-streams. When an elevated level is sustained, it contributes to obesity, suppresses our immune systems, causes osteoporosis, and interferes with lipid metabolism. And it keeps our blood pressure up.

Clearly, chronic stress—largely mediated by these two hormones—takes a significant toll on our bodies and contributes to the widespread problem of high blood pressure. It's something we need to understand, to identify in our individual lives, and to eliminate as much as possible. Not an easy task, but it can be done.

The first step is to take a long, hard look at ourselves. For those brave enough, you'll find a diagnostic tool at www.healthsceneinvestigation .com/files/2010/07/Percived-Stress-Scale.pdf (and yes, the misspelling "percived" is right for this address). This will get you started, and if you qualify as being "stressed out," you'll need to do something about it.

The treatment of chronic stress is beyond the scope of this book, but the cornerstone of that treatment is based on lifestyle evaluation and appropriate changes. Exercise, proper diet, adequate and sound sleep, attention to our relationships and to our emotional and spiritual lives. It's all tied together.

When managing your blood pressure, handling your stress level turns out to be really important. The good news: it *can* be done.

> "One way to get high blood pressure
> is to go mountain climbing over molehills."
> Earl Wilson (1907–1987)

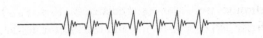

24

All You Need Is a Good Night's Sleep

You might be wondering why I'm including a discussion about sleep in a book on blood pressure. Not very long ago, I would have wondered the same thing. But as we learn more about hypertension and about the harmful effects of inadequate sleep, we are faced with the reality that they are connected. In fact, sleep disorders seem to be connected with just about everything. And most of those things are pretty bad.

The most important and most prevalent sleep disorder is called "obstructive sleep apnea" (OSA). Just what do we know about OSA?

The Centers for Disease Control (CDC) informs us that insufficient sleep is linked to the development of diabetes, cardiovascular disease (including high blood pressure, stroke, coronary artery disease, irregular heart rhythms such as atrial fibrillation, and hardening of the arteries), obesity, and depression. That's a long list, and should get our attention. Not only is OSA linked to these problems, but its presence makes the management of these disorders very difficult.

"Okay, Doc, but what's the connection between OSA and my elevated blood pressure?"

The answer to that question has everything to do with something we've already looked at—the *metabolic syndrome*. OSA appears to be a significant contributor to developing this cluster of related problems. Remember, this is a group of disorders including abdominal obesity, difficulties with handling our blood sugar, abnormal lipid levels, and high blood pressure. This last one is our concern here.

In addition to what the CDC has to say, multiple studies have demonstrated a consistent relationship between OSA and hypertension, coronary heart disease, heart failure, and irregular cardiac rhythms. The chief mechanism is felt to be due to a significant increase in sympathetic nervous activity during sleep. This results in an elevation in the chemicals that increase heart rate and raise blood pressure, and it's caused by a multitude of factors. These include low oxygen levels, elevations in carbon dioxide, and something called the "arousal response"—the fight-or-flight reaction to a perceived threat. If you can't breathe and suddenly wake up gasping for air, that might be a perceived threat.

The coexistence of OSA and hypertension is well established and is supported by several findings. In those of us without OSA, we experience a normal reduction in our blood pressure during sleep. Those with OSA don't have this dip, and blood pressures remain elevated during the entire night. We also know that individuals who don't have hypertension but develop OSA have an increased risk of developing high blood pressure. This is "dose-related" in that the worse the OSA, the greater the risk of hypertension. Mild OSA gives us twice the risk (compared to those without OSA) and severe OSA three times the risk. Finally, we see a definite relationship between OSA and "resistant hypertension"—the kind that's unresponsive to multiple medications and lifestyle changes. This is all too common, and we see it twice as frequently in those with OSA. Fortunately, when we treat the OSA, the hypertension usually improves.

Most people will see a reduction in their elevated blood pressure when their sleep disorder is corrected. The reduction is small—maybe 2 to 3 mm Hg—but even a lowering of this amount has been associated with a reduction in strokes, heart failure, and major cardiovascular events. Treating OSA makes a difference with your hypertension, and will help get and keep it under control. It needs to be noted that these findings have largely been based on the use of continuous positive airway pressure (CPAP) systems. Other therapies, such as oral appliances and even upper airway surgery, have not been well studied.

So we've established the connection between OSA and hypertension. Now we need to know a little more about OSA, how the diagnosis is made, and what kinds of treatments are available.

Simply stated, OSA is a common sleep-related *breathing* disorder, marked by recurrent episodes of apnea (you stop breathing) and variable degrees of upper airway obstruction during sleep. Well, maybe not so simple. The bottom line is excessive daytime sleepiness, snoring, and gasping or choking during sleep. Think that might be you? No? Maybe you need to ask your spouse or roommate. Fortunately, several screening tests are available that should raise some red flags if you do have OSA.

The first and easiest to complete is called the Sleep Apnea Clinical Score (SACS). It involves having someone measure the circumference of your neck. This is recorded in *centimeters* rather than inches because the smaller centimeter allows less error and variability in measurement. Then, the only things you need to know are whether you have high blood pressure (again, if you're on medication for this, you *have* high blood pressure) and whether you (1) snore or (2) have night-time choking or gasping. With these factors, you simply utilize a chart and find your score. A number of 15 or above indicates a high risk of OSA. This chart can be found at www.sleepmedicine.com/files/Forms/preoperative_questionnaire.pdf.

Another useful questionnaire is called the STOP BANG—an interesting acronym formed from the topics covered by the questions that are asked. It requires the following information:

Height in inches and centimeters: _____

Weight in pounds and kilograms: _____

Male/female: _____

Body Mass Index (BMI), which can be found in various tables, and you need to know your number): _____

Collar size of shirt in inches and centimeters: _____

Neck circumference in centimeters: _____

With that information in hand, you simply answer a series of questions, which you can find at www.stopbang.ca/screen.php.

Lastly, you'll find the "Berlin Questionnaire" at www.sleepapnea .org/assets/files/pdf/Berlin%20Questionnaire.pdf. This is a little more involved, but will help answer the question of your personal risk for this problem.

"So what do I do if one or all of these are positive?"

If that's the case, it's time to sit down and talk with your doctor. The next step would be a sleep study, either done in the comfort of your own home (this is becoming much more acceptable and increasingly available) or in a formal sleep lab, where you'll need to spend the night. This will provide a definitive diagnosis and guide your healthcare provider in offering an appropriate treatment plan.

Several effective options exist, but a word of caution. Surgery used to be the go-to treatment for OSA, but it's painful, costly, and not always effective. I ask my patients who have had the procedure (easily determined by a routine exam of the mouth and throat) if they are happy with the outcome. Did it work and would they do it over again? Fewer than half (probably closer to one in four) have been helped by the surgery, and fewer still would do it again. If I had to make a decision for myself, I would quickly opt for a nonsurgical approach, such as a CPAP machine or an oral appliance (called a mandibular advancement device), both of which help keep a person's airway open while they sleep.

In the meantime, if you think you might suffer from OSA, here are some tips for improving your sleep. Actually, this is good advice for all of us.

1. Go to bed and get up the same time each day, even on weekends and holidays. Establish a rhythm.

2. Don't eat within three to four hours of going to bed. And don't overeat.

3. Limit caffeine and nicotine—none within three to four hours of going to bed.

4. Limit alcohol consumption in the same way. Remember that alcohol *interferes* with efficient sleep; it doesn't help it.

5. Establish a routine before turning off the lights, and stick to it. Take a shower or bath, read a book, listen to soothing music.

6. Avoid TV or computer games just before going to bed. Not surprisingly, it appears this stimulation also interferes with your sleep. And for another "hot off the press" moment, it seems we need to avoid backlit reading devices (Kindle Fire, Nook) before turning out the lights. The light from these can stimulate certain parts of our brains, disrupting the normal

day/night cycle, and altering our cortisol levels. All of this may prolong the time it takes to get to sleep and lessen the quality of that sleep.

7. Create an environment conducive to restful sleep—cool, dark, quiet. Maybe consider a fan or other device to provide white noise to mask those thumps and bumps that might awaken you.

8. Quality pillows and mattresses (even sheets) are important and worth the investment.

9. Avoid long daytime naps—thirty minutes should be the max. Anything longer can make it harder to fall and stay asleep when you go to bed.

10. Regular physical exercise has been shown to help you fall asleep faster and to experience a deeper sleep. You'll need to experiment to determine how close to bedtime you can do this without being too energized.

For a lot of us, following these tips might be enough to help us sleep soundly and awake refreshed. For those who think they might have OSA, these will also be helpful, but you'll still need to complete a questionnaire, get tested, and find the best treatment plan for you.

And remember, you *do* need a good night's sleep.

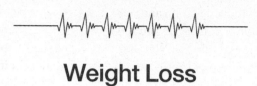

25

Weight Loss

Just how important is losing weight when it comes to lowering our blood pressure? It turns out to be pretty important. But from the outset, we need to acknowledge that it's hard to lose excess poundage in the first place, and then to keep it off is another challenge altogether. But it can be done, and any efforts here will be doubly rewarded.

So how is being overweight connected to our blood pressure? That continues to be a good question, though we have clear evidence that it is. You may have heard of the Framingham Heart Study, named after a town in eastern Massachusetts. This involved a large group of people followed for several decades, and looked at a bunch of different factors that affect our hearts and other aspects of our health. One of those factors was obesity. It turns out that excess body weight accounted for more than 25 percent of cases of high blood pressure in men and around 28 percent in women. In addition, about the same percentage of coronary artery disease in men was attributable to obesity and 15 percent in women. Those are big numbers, making this issue very significant.

Defining obesity and being overweight is fairly straightforward. These days we use our body mass index (BMI)—a calculation based on our height and weight—to determine where we are on a well-established and researched grid. If you don't know your number, there are many of these calculators online, and as we've already said, it's something you need to determine. Exceeding our ideal BMI places us at risk for several health-related problems, hypertension being one of them.

Several theories have been proposed for how obesity is related to high blood pressure. The first has to do with the hormone *insulin*. While critical in our handling of blood glucose, this simple chain of amino acids is not always our friend. While driving glucose into the cells of our bodies, it also stimulates the production and storage of fats, increases the storage of glucose in our livers, and raises our blood pressures. If we are overweight, there is an increased risk of *insulin resistance*. When this happens, the cells in our body don't respond as well to this hormone, more of it is produced, and all the bad things noted above get worse. And then we become diabetic, with all of its challenges.

Obstructive sleep disorders are also known to contribute to the development of hypertension. And we know that obesity is a risk factor for the onset and worsening of these disorders, including the sleep apnea syndrome. It's no coincidence that the first step in treating sleep disorders is to encourage weight loss.

Then there's the emerging field of *leptin* physiology. This is a protein that signals our brains when we've had plenty to eat, our fat stores are overloaded, and we need to cut back on our food. Some research indicates the clear association between the impairment of this negative feedback loop and the development of obesity, making this new frontier exciting and potentially very promising.

So while we might not know exactly *how* being overweight raises our blood pressure, we clearly know that when we lose weight, our pressures go down. But how much? In obese adults, both the systolic and diastolic pressures have been documented to fall by 1 mm Hg for each kilogram (2.2 pounds) of weight loss. To put that in perspective, losing eight to ten pounds is the equivalent of starting one blood pressure medication. That should get our attention. And again from the Framingham Study, if we are able to lose weight and *keep* it off—getting close to our ideal BMI and staying there—our chances of developing hypertension in the first place are reduced by more than 25 percent. That's a worthy goal.

Worthy, but difficult. It's hard to lose weight; it takes effort, motivation, and support. If weight loss were easy, it wouldn't be one of the most frequently searched topics on the Internet. But it can be done, and in many important ways, it will be worth it.

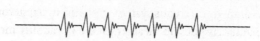

Have You Got a Light?
The Perils of Smoking

We know that smoking is one of the major risk factors for the development of heart disease, as well as emphysema and several deadly cancers. In fact, here's a sobering projection: Based on the number of current worldwide smokers (1.3 billion individuals, with 82 percent of these in developing countries), it is estimated that during this century, more than 1 billion people will suffer a tobacco-related death. Over 1 *billion.* That's something the makers of cigarettes should be proud of.

And here's something else they should be proud of: the percentage of monthly income that goes up in smoke in those developing countries. In Peru, where the monthly wage is around $268, smokers of one pack/day will spend almost *25 percent* of their money on cigarettes. In Pakistan, with an average monthly wage of $255, that percentage is only a few points less. Incredible, and troubling.

We also know that tobacco use is the most common cause of avoidable cardiovascular deaths. Stated another way, if people stopped smoking, the incidence of heart attacks, strokes, and heart failure would markedly fall. The key word here is *avoidable.* A lot of things will come our way that we won't be able to escape. But we want to give ourselves the best possible chance of avoiding the bad ones, and smoking cigarettes is not the way to do that. When it comes to preventive medicine, this is the low-hanging fruit. But boy is it hard to convince people to give up the habit. More about that a little later.

Just how does cigarette smoking raise our blood pressure, and how big is the effect? Let's start with how smoking affects our bodies.

With each drag, our nervous systems respond in dangerous ways: our heart rate immediately goes up, heart muscle contractility increases along with an increased cardiac demand for oxygen, and our blood pressures rise. These are the factors that are thought to be responsible for the increase in cardiovascular deaths. (The multiple carcinogens in tobacco smoke are the causes of lung cancer, but that's a different story.) The long-term rise in blood pressure is felt to be due to multiple factors, including the development of arterial stiffness caused by chronic smoking. The time it takes to start seeing these changes is unknown—maybe as little as one or two years—but the threshold number of cigarettes for developing this stiffness seems to be about fifteen per day.

One thing we *do* know is that with each cigarette, blood pressure can rise as much as 20 mm Hg. That's a lot, and it wreaks havoc within our vascular systems. The rise is temporary and begins to diminish over twenty to thirty minutes. This reaction seems to be most pronounced with the first cigarette of the day. We see this physical response in our clinic when performing physical exams for truck drivers seeking certification. To get in one last puff before their examination, they will stand by the front door until called. If their blood pressure is taken within thirty minutes of that cigarette, it will be elevated, sometimes to a level that disqualifies their certification. A little time in the exam room, and their pressure comes back down. Still a dangerous reality, and one that is frequently unappreciated. Sometimes, seeing these readings helps drive home the point to our patients that smoking in fact *does* elevate our blood pressures.

I mentioned "low hanging fruit" when it comes to guarding our health. There are so many reasons *not* to smoke or to quit if you do that this should be a no-brainer. Why in the world would anyone fall into the trap of this dangerous and filthy addiction? It's because of that—the *addiction*. If you smoke and think you're not addicted, you're wrong—maybe dead wrong.

"Frankie, you're wheezing and your X-ray shows some early pneumonia. We're going to start you on some antibiotics and an inhaler, but you've got to stop the smoking." I pointed to the Marlboros in the shirt pocket of this thirty-five-year-old man.

"Doc, I can't do it." Frankie had started smoking when he was thirteen, and his yellow-stained fingers loudly proclaimed his habit. But it was more than just a habit. "You know I've used drugs in the past, Doc. Clean now, thank heaven. You remember I almost died one night with a crack overdose."

I did remember. He had been carried into the ER by some "friends," dropped and abandoned at the ambulance entrance, and then been rushed into the cardiac room with no blood pressure and barely a pulse.

Frankie looked up and our eyes met. "You told me that night I had a choice to make—quit the cocaine or quit livin'. I knew you were right and made the choice to stop right then and there. Haven't messed with it since." He tapped his pack of cigarettes in his shirt pocket. "But I can't stop this. No matter how hard I try, I can't get off the cigarettes."

I had heard this before—too many times. Those who have fallen into the trap of substance abuse frequently tell me they were able to give up meth or cocaine, but they can't give up their cigarettes. It's more than just a habit. They're hooked.

It's the nicotine that gets them. Some abuse experts refer to it as the "perfect drug." It hits all the pleasure spots in our brains, creating a need for more and more of the drug. The makers of cigarettes have known this for decades, maybe from the moment the very first one was rolled. They've used this information to make sure their "clients" are addicted. Yes—addicted. If you smoke, that's you. Don't think so? Let me tell you about Myrtle Hawthorne.

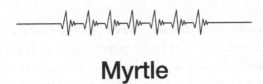

27

Myrtle

The ER—1979

"She's not breathing!"

The EMS stretcher crashed through the ambulance entrance, propelled by two red-faced paramedics.

"Cardiac!" our triage nurse called out, hurrying just steps ahead of them. She flung open the door and flipped a row of switches, flooding the room with bright overhead lights.

I knew the woman lying unresponsive on the gurney. Myrtle Hawthorne was fifty-two years old and a "frequent flyer" in the ER. She had a long history of emphysema, brought on by a thirty-year, two-pack-a-day history of cigarette smoking. When her chronic obstructive pulmonary disease (COPD) got bad enough, she would come to the ER for treatment.

"Just tune me up, Doc, and I'll be out of your hair," she'd say.

We were usually able to do that, and send her home after three or four hours of treatment. She received the same admonishment from me on every visit.

"Myrtle, you've got to stop smoking. Your lungs are only going to get worse, and one day we're not going to be able to 'tune you up.'"

Her plump, flushed face would break into a smile, and she would say, "I know, Doc. In fact, I quit a couple of weeks ago, but something happened at home and as we've already said, my nerves got tore up. Couldn't help it and I started back."

She may have paused with her smoking, but she had never quit. Each visit seemed worse than the one before, and it was getting harder to turn things around for her. As her motionless body flew by the nurses' station, I wondered if this was going to be that last time.

"Sorry, Dr. Lesslie," one of the paramedics said. "We couldn't get her intubated. Neck's too short, and I never saw her vocal cords."

He was using an ambu bag to ventilate this 5-foot, 225-pound woman. He was right; she had no neck and managing her airway was going to be difficult.

"That's okay, Jeff," I told him. "I know she's tough." Then turning to the nurse, "We need the airway tray, and open the tracheostomy kit too."

I didn't want to have to do a trach on Myrtle. In the best of circumstances it can be a difficult procedure, but with her peculiar anatomy, it might prove impossible. I wasn't sure I would be able to find the needed anatomical landmarks.

Fortunately—and with a great deal of luck—it didn't come to that. I was somehow able to snake an endotracheal tube through her vocal cords and into her trachea. The paramedic attached his ambu bag to the end of the tube, and I slowly forced air into her damaged lungs. There was a lot of resistance—her lungs were stiff and difficult to inflate. I glanced at the cardiac monitor. Her heart rate was thirty, dangerously low, and she still didn't have a pulse. Then forty, fifty, sixty.

"We've got something," the paramedic said, his fingers pressed over Myrtle's carotid artery.

"Seventy over fifty," the nurse relayed her blood pressure.

Things began to improve, and Myrtle started to make some respiratory attempts on her own. After an hour of ventilator support, a ton of medications, and divine intervention, she was stabilizing.

At one point her right hand flew up to the tube protruding from her mouth.

"Grab that," I told the nurse. "And secure her hands. We may lose her if she pulls that tube out."

An hour later, Myrtle was on her way to the ICU, still being bagged but responding more and moving all of her extremities. There was a reasonable chance she would survive.

Three days passed, and I was in the hospital cafeteria, getting some lunch. One of the ICU nurses walked past, and I asked, "How's Myrtle Hawthorne doing—the respiratory arrest we sent up a couple of days ago?"

"She's much better," the nurse answered. "We were able to move her to progressive care this morning."

"So she's off the ventilator?" I was surprised. Three days was a pretty fast turnaround.

"Yeah, but it wasn't easy. Right after she got to the unit, she grabbed her endotracheal tube and pulled it out. I don't know how you guys got her intubated 'cause the anesthesiologist couldn't. We had to get one of the surgeons to do a stat trach—barely in the nick of time. But she settled down and she's better. Already hand signaling for a cigarette."

I could imagine Myrtle doing just that and shook my head.

"Thanks. I'll try to get up to check on her."

It was another five days before I was able to make it to the fourth floor and the progressive care unit. The secretary at the nurses' station pointed down one of the long hallways to Myrtle's room, and I headed that direction.

I passed a couple of open doors and flinched as the acrid smell of cigarette smoke assaulted me. This was 1979, and we were just emerging from the Dark Ages. It was still possible to smoke in the hospital as long as you had the written permission of your doctor. A lot of the physicians on staff didn't want the hassle of dealing with irate family members or begging patients, and they routinely wrote "Smoking Permitted" on their patient's chart. The Dark Ages.

I stopped at room 432 and checked the name tag on the door: *Myrtle Hawthorne—Dr. Osterman.*

It was a semiprivate room, but Myrtle was the only patient. I pushed the door open, stepped in, and pulled aside the curtain surrounding her bed. A cloud of smoke billowed toward me and I almost gagged.

Myrtle was lying comfortably, head raised as she watched the wall-mounted television at the foot of her bed. She turned to me, smiled, and gave me a slow, circular wave with one hand. With the other, she carried a smoking cigarette to the tracheostomy hole in her neck, placed it in the dark cavity, and took a long, deep drag. Smoke curled from the hole and escaped through her nostrils.

I just stood there. Then I turned and walked out of the room.

28

You Gotta Know Your Numbers

The Sentinel

"Robert...Frank Jamison here. I need a little help."

"Sure, Frank. What's going on?"

Frank was a local family practitioner, one of the first in this town. Now in his eighties, he continued to practice full-time, seeing patients in his office five-and-a-half days a week, and always coming to the ER if one of them needed to be admitted. It didn't matter if it was in the dead of night or the dead of winter—Frank Jamison would take care of "his people." He had seen it all and then some. When he asked for help, I paid attention.

"I'm going to send Peg Anderson over to the ER. She's one of my nurses, and I'd like for you to take a look at her. See what you think and let me know."

"I'll be glad to, Frank. What's her problem?"

"Not exactly sure." He paused, and I could imagine him scratching the top of his head and scrunching his eyes. "Something's just not right with her this afternoon. She'll tell you about it. And don't forget to call."

He hung up, and I handed the phone to the secretary. Lori Davidson, our triage nurse, walked past the nurses' station.

"Lori, that was Dr. Jamison. He's sending one of his nurses over for us to see. Peg Anderson, I think he said."

"I know Peg. She and I are about the same age. We went to nursing school together. She's okay, isn't she?"

"I don't know. Just be on the lookout for her. I'm sure she'll be coming through triage here in a few minutes."

Fifteen minutes later, Lori led her thirty-eight-year-old friend through the triage door, past the nurses' station, and into room 5. Peg didn't appear to be in any distress as she walked past, and even managed a smile—not always easy to do when you're a patient in the ER.

Lori stood by her stretcher and the two friends were chatting as I entered the room. "Okay, Peg," I said. "Tell me what's going on. You've got Dr. Jamison a little concerned."

She shook her head and smiled again. "You know Dr. Frank. Always worried about the least little thing."

"And he's usually right to be worried," Lori gently asserted.

"Well, it was just something funny," Peg began. "I had just gotten back from my lunch break and was checking on one of our patients. I started having this sharp pain right above my eye, and for a second my vision got a little blurred. Just for a second, and then it was back to normal. I had been talking with the patient and tried to say something, but the words wouldn't come out. That scared me a little. It only lasted for ten, maybe fifteen seconds, but I've never experienced anything like it. I knew what I wanted to say, but I couldn't form the words."

"So that lasted about fifteen seconds?" I asked.

Peg nodded.

"And what about the headache—the pain behind your eye? Is it still there? Still as bad?"

"It's still there but not nearly as bad. Maybe a one or two out of ten."

I noticed that her left upper eyelid was drooping. Just a little, but definitely there. I asked her about it. Her hand flew to her face and she blinked several times.

"I've never noticed anything like that before." She turned to Lori and raised her eyebrows.

Lori studied her face and said, "Yes, it's drooping. But only a little."

Peg turned to me, her face flushing. "What do you think that means?"

"I'm not sure yet, but we're going to put all this together. Let's go over your medical history."

I scanned through the information on her chart. No allergies and her only listed medication was lisinopril 20 mgs—a blood pressure medication. Her temperature was normal and her heart rate was fine at sixty-two. But her blood pressure was 158/100.

"Tell me about your blood pressure, Peg."

"I've had hypertension since right after nursing school. Not bad, but high enough to be on medication. I'm just not very good at taking it."

"Did you take it this morning? Or yesterday?"

Peg sighed. "I don't think I've taken it in a couple of days. It doesn't cause any side effects or anything, I just forget to take it. Don't tell Dr. Frank, though. He gets on me all the time about it."

Other than the drooping eyelid, the remainder of Peg Anderson's examination was completely normal. I was worried about something going on in her head and asked about any family history of strokes or neurologic problems. Nothing, just some heart disease and a few relatives with high blood pressure.

"I'd like to get a scan of your brain," I told her.

This time she turned pale and stammered, "I'm working the next two days, but sometime Thursday should be okay."

I put a hand on her shoulder. "We need to get a scan right now."

Forty-five minutes later, one of the radiologists called me.

"Robert, this Peg Anderson of yours. Looks like she's got a good-sized berry aneurysm sitting in the left front of her brain—about half an inch in diameter. May even have been leaking a little. What kind of symptoms has she been having?"

I described her complaints and findings. "It sounded like it might have been a sentinel bleed," I told him. "And if there *has* been some bleeding, I guess that was her warning."

"She's mighty lucky," he said. "You just don't know when these things are going to burst, and then it's lights-out."

I handed the phone to the secretary and stood there. Peg Anderson *was* lucky. And this was pretty scary. No family history of anything like this, and her only risk factor was high blood pressure. But that was enough. She had been given a warning—this "sentinel bleed"—which was more than most people with this type of aneurysm receive.

"Can you get the neurosurgeon on call on the phone?" I asked the secretary. "And then Dr. Frank."

29

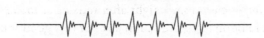

The Fine Print:
Making Sense of Those Labels

Reading nutritional food labels may not be as enjoyable as reading a *New York Times* bestseller, but you just might learn some interesting things, improve your and your family's health, and if done correctly, *not* tick off the store manager.

That's right—there's an acceptable way to do this and a way…Well, I'll just give you some advice. My wife suggested I use my smartphone to gather information for this chapter. Simply take some pictures of labels and study them at home at my leisure. Not going to happen. It seems most if not all grocery stores frown upon shoppers taking pictures. Take my word for this and don't try it. I was glad I had a clipboard with pre-printed info sheets and could study boxes and cans and make notes of all the numbers. It was a little cumbersome, and I still had some 'splainin' to do, but it worked.

Before I share some of the things I learned, let's take a look at a "nutritional food label" and try to understand what information it contains. The Food and Drug Administration has a great website for this at www.fda .gov/Food/IngredientsPackagingLabeling/LabelingNutrition/ucm274593 .htm. Below is one of their examples and a good place to begin.

Nutrition Facts

Serving Size 2/3 cup (55g)
Servings Per Container About 8

Amount Per Serving

Calories 230   Calories from Fat 72

                                              % Daily Value*

Total Fat 8g	**12%**
Saturated Fat 1g	**5%**
Trans Fat 0g	
Cholesterol 0mg	**0%**
Sodium 160mg	**7%**
Total Carbohydrate 37g	**12%**
Dietary Fiber 4g	**16%**
Sugars 1g	
Protein 3g	

Vitamin A	10%
Vitamin C	8%
Calcium	20%
Iron	45%

* Percent Daily Values are based on a 2,000 calorie diet.
Your daily value may be higher or lower depending on
your calorie needs.

	Calories:	2,000	2,500
Total Fat	Less than	65g	80g
Sat Fat	Less than	20g	25g
Cholesterol	Less than	300mg	300mg
Sodium	Less than	2,400mg	2,400mg
Total Carbohydrate		300g	375g
Dietary Fiber		25g	30g

Let's start with "Serving Size." This is really important and frequently overlooked. It can be tricky, and I've misread this myself, on more than one occasion. In this example, the serving size is 2/3 of a cup. It's worth the time to take out a measuring cup and see how much we're talking about. If it's breakfast cereal, I bet you're eating a lot more than 2/3 of a cup. The tricky part for me is when the serving size is given in ounces or teaspoons or tablespoons. You have to pay attention. These sizes make a big difference in calorie counts, fat grams, and carbs.

Let's go to "Calories." This is straightforward, but you have to remember the serving size. If this example is for a breakfast cereal and you're eating two cups of it, that's more than twice the amount of calories listed. Simple math, but you have to pay attention. As for the "Calories from Fat," you don't have to pay much attention to this if you're on a low-carb diet.

While we're talking about calories, here's a sobering thought. It's generally accepted that if you take in 3,000 more calories than you burn, you will gain one pound. In other words, you have to burn 3,000 calories to lose one pound. Twenty minutes on a treadmill at 3.7 mph at an incline of 5 degrees burns about 150 calories. One 12-ounce can of regular soda contains 140 calories. Go figure.

Now we move on to "Total Fat." This area of the label breaks down the fat content of a product. This particular label lists only saturated fat and trans fat, while others will break it down further to tell us how much of the total fat is mono or polyunsaturated. The trans-fat number here is 0 grams, which is good. This type of fat should be disappearing from the US marketplace. Bear in mind that the FDA does not require listing an amount if the trans-fat content is less than 0.5 grams in a serving, so this unnatural and deadly grease can still be present and add up. For the most part, take the "Total Fat" and subtract the "Saturated" variety. That leaves us with the unsaturated and healthier kinds. Remember, we need to work on reducing the saturated fat in our diets.

Next we see the "Cholesterol" content of this food. We should limit this in our diets, but keep in mind it's not so much the cholesterol we take in that drives up the level in our body. It's several factors, including our individual genetic makeup, the amount of carbs we eat, and the amount of exercise we get.

The "Sodium" (salt) content, what we're really interested in here, is important for all of us, especially if our blood pressure is high or even borderline. Actually, *all* of us need to limit this mineral because of its harmful effects. That's difficult, because it finds its way into many of our processed foods. The American Heart Association currently recommends an intake of less than 1500 mgs/day. With our example, you can see how this adds up. Later, we'll take a more in-depth look at the impact of sodium on our blood pressures.

Now the "Total Carbohydrate" numbers. This is another place where we really need to pay attention. The low-carb approach targets 60 grams as a limit. I think this number can be bumped to 100, but as you can see, this example shows 37 grams. That's typical for a lot of cereals, breads, and other processed grains. And with only one serving, you're well on your way to the daily max.

"Dietary Fiber" is important, and remember the recommended daily amount of 25 grams for women and 38 for men. Most nutrition experts will refer to "net carbs." This is calculated by subtracting the fiber amount from the total carbohydrate. (Some recommend subtracting half of the fiber.) The more fiber in a food, the lower its glycemic index and the less impact it will have on your blood sugar.

Next we see "Sugars." This is the total amount of natural sugars (as found in fruit and milk, for example) along with any added sugars. It's the added ones you need to pay attention to, and these can be found in the "Ingredients" section, which usually appears on product packaging somewhere near the "Nutrition Facts." Added sugars can include corn syrup, high-fructose corn syrup, fruit juice concentrate, maltose, dextrose, sucrose, and even honey and maple syrup. All of these add carbs to our diet and are largely unneeded.

A couple of points: When we study these food labels, we're probably holding in our hands something processed—something we need to eliminate as much as possible from our diets. And the ingredients list on a food label works just like the ingredients list on a pet food label—contents are listed in descending order by weight. Something to keep in mind for you and your pet.

The amount of "Protein" listed is just that and is of concern if you have to limit your intake, usually because of significant kidney problems. It's also of interest because of the places you find—or don't find—this essential building block.

That leaves us with the percentage of recommended daily allowances for various vitamins and minerals. I don't pay much attention to this since it really doesn't enter into my equation for determining the healthiness of a particular food. For instance, in our example, you would have to eat almost 7 cups of this stuff to achieve 100 percent of your daily vitamin A needs. Yet, you may find this information interesting.

Now that we have a handle on reading a nutritional label, brace yourselves—the FDA is proposing to revise it. You can find an example on the FDA website listed earlier in this chapter, and it actually makes a lot of sense. The important things are emphasized and the not-so-important are minimized.

I mentioned my fact-finding trip to the grocery store. In addition to learning that cameras aren't allowed, I found the following to be of interest:

- A lot of us eat salads and salad dressings. All of these dressings contain fats, but mostly of the healthy kind. You have to watch the amounts (most list 2 tablespoons as one serving) so the calories can quickly add up. The lowest in carb content are blue cheese (1 gram per serving) followed by ranch (1 to 2 grams).

- You have to pay attention to the "lite" dressings. Sounds healthy, but they take out some of the fat and add a lot of sugar. Some of these have 16 to 18 grams/serving.

- All of our breakfast cereals are loaded with carbs, and many have added sugars—especially those we feed to our children.

- Check the sugar contents of "healthy" and "all-natural" fruit drinks. And bring your insulin.

- As a general rule, anything labeled "all-natural" should be carefully scrutinized.

Make it a habit to read those labels. And just remember, as someone once said, "If it comes in a can, box, wrapper, or through a fast-food window, it's probably going to eventually kill you."

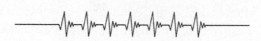

30

Complementary and Alternative Medicine (CAM)

"Doc, my cousin says that if you drink a quart of prune juice every morning, your blood pressure will go down. What do you think?"

He seemed serious, so I needed to give him a serious answer, if there was one.

We're frequently asked about alternative treatments for many common ailments, especially what we think about their effectiveness. It all depends, but first let's define these terms.

Alternative medicine refers to the use of a nonmainstream approach *in place of* conventional, mainstream medicine. *Complementary medicine* refers to using a nonmainstream approach *along with* mainstream medicine.

A true alternative approach to a medical problem—for instance, treating bacterial pneumonia with poultices—is not very common. It's much more likely we'll combine nonmainstream and conventional treatments if we're convinced of the effectiveness of both.

For our discussion here, we'll use the acronym CAM, which stands for "complementary and alternative medicine." It encompasses all the various nonmainstream treatments available to us. The margins begin to blur a little with the passage of time. What was earlier considered to be CAM has become more conventional. A few examples are the utilization of fish oil in the treatment of elevated triglyceride levels and niacin to elevate low

HDL levels. Prior to that would be the native Peruvians' discovery of the medicinal use of the bark of the cinchona tree. It found widespread use as a treatment for malaria (quinine) and a cardiac medicine (quinidine), variations of which are still in use today.

How common is the use of CAM therapies in the United States? It appears that one in five of us will employ some form of this treatment, with the choices including acupuncture, ayurveda (a system of Hindu traditional medicine), homeopathy, Chinese or Oriental medicine, chiropractic, massage, body movement therapies, tai chi, yoga, dietary supplements, herbal medicine, biofeedback, electromagnetic therapy, qigong (balancing your chi or "life energy"), meditation, hypnosis, and even art, dance, and music. Whew.

In the US, the most frequently used CAM therapies (in descending order) are: herbal remedies, breathing meditation, other forms of meditation, chiropractic manipulation, yoga, diet-based therapy, progressive relaxation, and megavitamin therapy. Interestingly, the British National Health Service lists their three most commonly employed CAM therapies as acupuncture, aromatherapy, and chiropractic. I wonder if that's a spinal manipulation with a needle in your ear and a rose in your nose.

The problem we face with CAM therapies is determining their effectiveness and safety. We have the same dilemma with our conventional treatments, whether they be pharmaceutical, surgical, or other (such as radiation therapy). It all comes down to performing rigorous and reproducible research. That takes money, and frequently a lot of it. Our pharmaceutical companies have it to spend, and they fund much (many think *too* much) of our ongoing medical research. They need to prove their latest medicines will work and are safe so they can get them to the market.

As you can imagine, there's probably not a lot of research going on with ayurveda or regarding the use of dance for depression. When it does happen, most studies fail to demonstrate any beneficial outcomes with many CAM therapies. There have been a couple of noteworthy exceptions. The practice of tai chi has been shown to significantly reduce the incidence of falls among our elderly, probably due to better conditioning and balance. And several types of acupuncture have proven effective for selected conditions, including low-back pain and migraine headaches. Probably not better than conventional treatments and usually more expensive, but it seems to work. With the passage of time, many of these CAM therapies, or elements of them, may merge into the conventional.

Until then, I'm going to keep an open mind but rely on reputable journal reports and the results of well-designed and large studies. If you're considering a CAM therapy, talk with your physician. If she tries to discourage you and you forge ahead anyway, just be sure to let her know. After all, that next tree you chew on may be the secret to everlasting youth, or at least a cure for baldness.

And no, a quart of prune juice every morning is not going to help your blood pressure. But you'd better stay near a bathroom.

However, there are some CAM therapies that might be useful in our battle against hypertension, and we'll look at some of those.

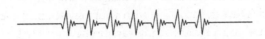

31

CAM: What Really Works?

Since a lot of us are using some form of complementary or alternative medicine, it's important to ask what really works. As we mentioned in the last chapter, CAM can take several forms, such as vitamins and herbal supplements or chiropractic and mind-body therapies. Let's start with the herbal things.

It turns out that the majority of us—somewhere north of 65 percent of US adults—are taking *something*. And we're spending more than six billion dollars a year. Here's a list of the most popular natural products and the estimated percentage of adults taking them. You'll probably note a few you're taking yourself, maybe upon the advice of your physician.

Fish oil—37.4 percent
Echinacea—19.8 percent
Flaxseed oil—15.9 percent
Ginseng—14.1 percent
Ginkgo biloba—11.3 percent
Garlic—11.0 percent

Coenzyme Q10—8.7 percent
Fiber or psyllium—6.6 percent
Green tea pills—6.3 percent
Cranberry—6.0 percent
Saw palmetto—5.1 percent
Soy supplements—5.0 percent

In addition to these top-sellers, the shelves of our grocery and health-food stores are piled high with a wide assortment of exotic-sounding products, each touting their special abilities in improving just about every aspect of our lives. We won't be able to cover them all, but if you want some information about a particular supplement, here are a few reliable resources:

www.consumerlab.com
www.ods.od.nih.gov
www.dsld.nlm.nih.gov/dsld/index.jsp
www.nccam.nih.gov/health/herbsataglance.htm
(I highly recommend this last site.)

Herbal Products and Supplements

What we find when we study the evidence is that there are a few herbal supplements or vitamins that might be of use, a few that are clearly dangerous, and a whole bunch in the middle. We're still learning about this and trying to sort it all out. For now, though, we're interested in what might be of benefit with the lowering of blood pressure. Let's see what we know.

Garlic. In addition to repelling vampires, there is some evidence that garlic may lower blood pressure. The degree of reduction is small—only a few mm Hg—and the amount needed is about 2 grams a day of the powder or extract. If you want to give this a try, it may take as much as twelve weeks before results will be seen.

Chocolate. We're talking about dark chocolate here, and maybe as much as 50 grams a day. That amount can result in a significant increase in calories, while potentially lowering your BP by only 2 to 3 mm Hg. It does this by affecting certain enzymes in the kidney and by increasing levels of nitric oxide that dilate blood vessels. Though most forms of chocolate contain large amounts of sugar as well as caffeine, the emerging evidence regarding the health benefits of dark chocolate is largely positive.

Fish oil (omega-3 fatty acids). In addition to lowering triglycerides, fish oil can help lower blood pressure in many people. The reduction is going to be small, and a higher dose may be required than is normally recommended for lipid management. But this is worth a try, since the downside is very small.

Magnesium. This is one of our essential minerals, and though we don't need a lot of it, when we're deficient, we can see our blood pressures go up. If we replace the deficit, our BP comes down. It's a potent vasodilator and can lower our pressure by as much as 3 to 4 mm Hg.

Vitamin D. The evidence favoring this vitamin in the treatment of high blood pressure is similar to the evidence we have for magnesium. Low levels of vitamin D are associated with hypertension, while returning those levels to normal will usually lower that person's BP. It's easy to have this level checked, and most of us will need a supplement to get and keep us in the normal range. The correct amount is currently the source of much debate, but I recommend my patients take 1000 to 2000 units of vitamin D3 each day. That's what I take myself.

Coenzyme Q10. This substance is also known as *ubiquinone* because of it's ubiquitous distribution in the natural world. It seems to be everywhere and in many foods. There is good evidence to support its use in congestive heart failure, type 2 diabetes, migraine headaches, and even Parkinson's disease. Some experts recommend it to help prevent and treat the muscle pain associated with statin drugs.

Regarding our blood pressures, several large studies have demonstrated a reduction in systolic/diastolic pressures of as much as 16/9 mm Hg with Coenzyme Q10 alone. That's impressive and as good as or better than adding a blood pressure medication. The doses used in these studies were between 60 and 120 mgs, given up to three times a day. That sounds like a lot, but no serious side effects were noted. If you try this, you might start at 60 mgs twice a day and monitor your BP. You can always add more.

In summary, if you have high blood pressure, you can safely consider any of these supplements. However, the best current evidence supports the use of CoQ10 and dark chocolate, so that's where I'd put my money.

Mind-Body Techniques

Now about mind-body approaches. These interventions focus on our ability to learn how to relax, slow our heart rates, and lower our blood pressures. Easier said than done. But we have some interesting evidence to support several techniques.

Qigong. This is a traditional Chinese medicine technique that incorporates breathing, movement, and meditation. The amount of blood pressure reduction is impressive—as much as 17/10 mm Hg. If you want to try this, you'll need to find a local instructor for the best and safest results.

Slow, controlled breathing. Sounds simple enough, and it is. It also works. We know that slowed breathing can reduce the activity of our sympathetic nervous system—the pathway responsible for our fight-or-flight reactions. The key is to achieve the correct level and rate of breathing and to maintain it. Interestingly, the FDA has approved at least one over-the-counter device to help you do this, and information can be found at www.resperate.com.

Meditation. While there has been some controversy surrounding this topic, the main idea here is to learn to relax and reduce the emotional influences that might be raising our heart rate and blood pressure. There is good information to indicate that such relaxation is helpful. There's also emerging evidence indicating that prayer may very well have the same effects.

Physical exercise. We've talked about the importance of physical activity in maintaining our health and lowering our blood pressure. The best evidence of this exists for dynamic and aerobic exercise. Dynamic, or isotonic, refers to the regular, purposeful movement of joints and large muscle groups. (Whereas *isometric* exercise involves the static contraction of muscles without joint movement.) This would include such things as weight lifting and push-ups. Aerobic exercises include such things as high-speed walking, jogging, running, swimming, and even dancing. All of these activities will help lower your blood pressure.

Many of our hypertensive patients also have joint problems, involving the back, hips, and knees. These people naturally find it difficult to do any of the above exercises and may be limited to slow walking, if even that. They need to be encouraged to find some form of aerobic activity that will improve their cardiac health and lower their blood pressures. The good news here is that upper-limb aerobic exercise will help do just that. The best activity turns out to be "arm cycling," using a stationary device. If you've never tried this, be forewarned. This is a tough exercise, and needs gradual and careful progression. But it can lower your blood pressure by as much as 7/6 mm Hg.

And lastly, how many of us have a lowly spring-loaded handgrip device hiding somewhere in our home or office? We probably bought it thinking it would be a good way to relieve stress while on the phone, in front of our computer, or sitting and reading. It turns out that it *does* relieve stress. And if used vigorously for about thirty minutes each week, it can lower your blood pressure by as much as 13/8 mm Hg! Who would have thunk it? That's the same as your lisinopril tablet. But the evidence is there, and if your experience is only half that, it's still something to strongly think about doing.

So as far as the mind-body techniques we have to choose from, the best choices are qigong (if interested and you can find an instructor), slow-breathing techniques, some form of meditation and regular prayer, and physical activity. And don't forget to start those handgrip exercises, though it will be hard to do that and eat chocolate at the same time.

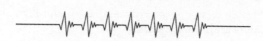

32

CAM: Where You Can Save Your Money

It was P.T. Barnum who said, "There's a sucker born every minute." I think it's much more frequent than that.

We all make poor decisions with how we spend our money (I know I do), and it seems we're always looking for the easiest way to deal with difficult problems (I do that too). It's especially true when it comes to our health and, in this instance, when it comes to trying to lower our blood pressure. We know what it will take—exercise, salt restriction, weight loss—but none of that is much fun. Give me a pill or two and I'll be happy. As P.T. also knew, there would always be folks around who'd be only too happy to provide you with those pills—at a price.

So how do we avoid those folks, and how do we make right decisions when it comes to spending our money on our health? In the last chapter, we considered some of the complementary and alternative medicine options that would be reasonable to try. There's good evidence to support their ability to lower your blood pressure—maybe by only a few mm Hg, but those add up.

In the next chapter, we'll look at those things we need to avoid for health reasons. These are the herbal remedies that have been shown to damage various organs and cause a lot of different and significant problems.

In this chapter, we're going to consider the CAMs you should also avoid, not because of the harm they may do to your health but because of the harm they may do to your wallet. For these CAMs, there is little if any evidence that they are beneficial. This will end up being the majority of the products in the marketplace, so I'm going to offend some people. But my goal here is to save you time and money.

Herbal Products and Supplements

Let's start with the herbal products and supplements. The list of substances claiming to help lower blood pressure is extensive, and we'll be able to cover only some of these. If you're tempted to take something that's not mentioned here, check it out before doing so. Remember, none of these herbals has any hard proof to substantiate their claims. There might be some anecdotal claims, and maybe some weak observational studies, but unless rigorous controlled studies have been performed, their benefits remain unproved.

Astragalus. Commonly used in traditional and contemporary Chinese medicine, and available in capsules, teas, and various extracts. It's also known as *Bei qi, huang qi, and milk vetch.* There are no proven benefits and it might in fact suppress your immune system.

Cat's Claw. Lots of claims, but no proven benefits.

Cinnamon. Several recent medical articles have reported potential benefits with regular consumption of this spice, but as of now, there's no solid evidence. We'll have to wait and see.

Cardamom. Another spice with unproved potential.

Ginseng. This is a commonly used herb, but claims of lowering blood pressure have never been substantiated.

Licorice root. This actually has the opposite effect—it *raises* your blood pressure by affecting your adrenal glands which then act on your kidneys.

Sandalwood. Again, many claims but no proof.

Hawthorn berry. Same as for sandalwood.

Myrrh. That's right, the stuff carried by the three wise men. While most of its claims are as an antiseptic and anti-fungal, its benefits are alleged only. No proof. Stick with gold and frankincense.

And you've got to be a little suspicious about herbs with names like *slippery elm, solid bone, snake weed, Solomon's seal,* and *zizyphus.*

Again, the list of herbal remedies with claims of lowering blood pressure is lengthy, with the overwhelming majority being unfounded. This is a good place to save your money.

Mind-Body Techniques

Now about those mind-body techniques. We know that aerobic and dynamic exercise works, as does the spring-loaded handgrip. And we know that certain types of meditation are effective. But what *doesn't* work? Or what hasn't yet been proven to be effective?

Biofeedback techniques. While there is some evidence that these might produce slight reductions in blood pressure, the results of large studies are not consistent, the cost is significant, and long-term management remains a problem.

Yoga. The practice of yoga has been highly touted of late, both as a stress-reducer and as a way of staying physically fit. Originating in ancient India, its goal is to achieve cessation of mental activity (I accomplished that with ease during some of my college courses) and the attainment of a state of superior consciousness (haven't been there yet). There have been claims that practicing this will lower your blood pressure, but no reliable confirmation exists. Any reasonable studies undertaken have yielded mixed results, so save your money.

Stress management and other relaxation techniques. These come in many shapes and sizes, and while some may someday prove to be helpful for the treatment of hypertension, no solid evidence currently exists to support their use. Interestingly, one study that utilized the music of Mozart for twelve sessions of twelve minutes each found a reduction in systolic blood pressure. Unfortunately, and maybe predictably, when these BPs were measured one and three months later, there was no difference from baseline. Yet, relaxing music may have its place here. Led Zeppelin not so much.

Acupuncture. For decades now, there have been claims that acupuncture can lower blood pressure. As you can imagine, it's hard to have truly "blinded" clinical trials to determine its effectiveness compared to other forms of treatment, making its study difficult. Yet, some evidence exists that certain types of acupuncture, in the right hands, can be helpful. This remains to be seen, and until that time comes—if it does—you should save your money with this one too.

Gemstone therapy. I came across this fascinating therapy to treat blood pressure. In addition to lowering your BP, it's possible to improve your physical and emotional health by applying specific gemstones and crystals to various parts of your body. (What was it that P.T. had to say?)

Amber—lifts emotional heaviness, promoting happiness

Apatite—helps communication and fights viruses (now *that's* an impressive stone)

Green aventurine—heals minor illnesses. If you have something more serious going on, you will need to add *emerald* or *frosted quartz.*

Carnelian—stops wheezing

Green fluorite—helps with PMS and menopause

Mexican onyx—helps one sleep better

Sapphire—useful for mental clarity and helping one clear "mental garbage"

I wonder if I can find my pet rock from the seventies. Who knows what wondrous things might be possible.

So there's a list of things to avoid and ways to save your money. We'll keep an eye on some potentially promising techniques, such as acupuncture and maybe some of the stress-reducing maneuvers. They may yet prove to be helpful. Carnelian stones for your wheezing and asthma? Stick with your inhalers.

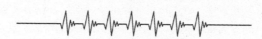

33

CAM: Things You Need to Avoid

While the many complementary alternative medicine activities and herbals are largely innocent—simply wasting your time and money—several are dangerous and need to be avoided. Some in this category have been removed from the marketplace, while others persist in being available to unsuspecting buyers. You may have read about some of these, but we need to continue to be keenly aware of their dangers.

The first herbal in this list is *ephedra*. Also marketed as *ma huang*, this substance has been touted for weight loss and athletic enhancement. In fact, it has been found to *increase* blood pressure and *cause* heart attacks, strokes, and seizures. In addition, it frequently causes psychiatric and gastrointestinal complications. Several deaths have been directly attributable to this herbal product, prompting the FDA to ban it in 2004. There remains some concern that it can still be found in various herbal combinations, since there is little quality assurance for most of these products.

Several supplements have been associated with liver damage, at times proving fatal:

chaparral leaf (greasewood,
creosote bush)
jin bu huan
germander

kava (a popular and dangerous
herb)
mistletoe
skullcap
pennyroyal

Some herbal products have been found to demonstrate active hormonal activity, such as estrogen and testosterone, a potential problem for young people approaching or experiencing puberty, as well as those of us who are being treated for various types of hormone-dependent or sensitive cancers.

Estrogenic effects

alfalfa	red clover
aniseed	saw palmetto
black cohosh	wild carrot
ginseng	

Other hormonal effects

bayberry and licorice (can affect the adrenal gland)
horseradish (may suppress the thyroid gland)

And since our discussion here is about controlling our blood pressures, several herbs have been shown to elevate our BP, the opposite of what we're working hard to do:

bayberry	ginger
broom	ginseng
blue cohosh	licorice
coltsfoot	

One final concern is the problem of herb-drug interactions—the effects herbs can have on important prescription medicines we might be taking. This is especially perplexing for physicians since many of our patients don't consider vitamins and herbal remedies as being significant enough to mention to their healthcare provider, and they don't. Some of the more important interactions include the following:

Ginkgo biloba (taken to purportedly enhance memory) has significant anticlotting properties, including deactivation of platelets. When combined with Coumadin (warfarin) or aspirin, serious bleeding complications can arise.

Most of us have heard of the problems with *grapefruit juice* and certain medications. When taken with some of the calcium channel blockers (which we'll talk about in chapter 41), the activity of the hypertensive medication can be increased and a dangerously low blood pressure can develop. This can lead to a lot of problems including falls, strokes, and even heart attacks.

Saint-John's-wort is supposed to be helpful in the treatment of depression and a lot of us have tried it. When taken with a prescription antidepressive medication, the "serotonin syndrome" can develop, resulting in sweating, rapid heartbeat, kidney failure, and seizures. Nothing fun here.

There are many documented interactions and problems with the use of some of the commonly available herbal products. We need to do a little research (take a look at those websites I listed a couple of chapters back) and always be cautious with what we put into our bodies.

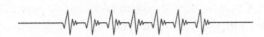

34

CAM: A Realistic and Workable Approach

We've covered a lot about complementary and alternative medicine, and taken a look at some of the things that work, some that don't, and what you must stay away from. Now we're going to try to pull all of this together and make sense out of what we now know.

There's one thing we can hang our hats on—this whole area will be changing. We will learn more about these approaches, and some of the seemingly useful strategies may be moved to the "don't waste your money" column. At the same time, I hope we will see the development of additional CAMs that will clearly help in the management of our blood pressures, and these may come from places we didn't expect and couldn't envision. That's the exciting part of all this.

But the confusing and sometimes frustrating part now is, "What am I supposed to do with all this information? Which of these ideas should I incorporate into my daily regimen as I battle hypertension, and when should I do it?"

Take heart. We have some help answering these questions, and it comes from a reputable and trustworthy source, the American Heart Association (AHA). They have studied this issue and come up with a comprehensive but straightforward approach to help us incorporate CAM into our treatment of hypertension.

We're going to go through these steps (relax, there are only three of them) and sort out the things we need to know. First and most importantly, when these guidelines state "alternative approach," we will be talking only about the things that have been proven to work. Regarding the advice of the AHA, these will largely be mind-body maneuvers, but I will suggest we include the other things that will probably help, such as some of the herbal supplements and vitamins we discussed earlier.

Step 1: Prehypertension

This step guides us in our approach to individuals with prehypertension, which means their blood pressure is above normal but not yet in the hypertensive range. We also know that most people in this stage will go on to develop full-blown hypertension. The AHA recommends a good diet (including significant salt restriction) and aggressive lifestyle changes—exercise, weight loss, no smoking. At the same time, CAM can be started and continued for up to a year. If blood pressure remains less than 140/90, we can continue doing what we're doing. If it's been a year and our BP hasn't improved, it's time to move to Step 2 and possibly begin medication. During this one-year prehypertension trial period, it's okay to change around some of our CAMs and try something we haven't done before.

Let's say we've tried things for a year and our BP remains elevated. Now what? It's time to move on to Step 2.

Step 2: Untreated Hypertension

If we still want to avoid medication and our BP is in the range without any evidence of heart, kidney, or neurological problems, we can start or continue an alternative approach. The AHA would allow six to twelve months for this, depending on any risks for cardiovascular disease (smoking, family history of heart disease, elevated lipids). Once again, if our pressure is less than 140/90 at the end of this period, we can keep on keeping on. If not, it's time to add drug therapy. It can't be stressed enough that aggressive lifestyle changes are essential if this strategy is to be successful. And again, we can adjust our chosen CAMs and change them around if desired.

If our blood pressure is high enough that we begin to see evidence of target organ damage, we will definitely need to start medication. The AHA guideline states that we can *add* CAM at this point if desired. The reason for doing this would be to reduce the chances of having to add another blood pressure medication or increase the dosage of what we're already taking. If we meet our blood pressure goal, we should continue what we're doing. If not, an adjustment in medication will be necessary.

Step 3: Treated Hypertension

If our blood pressure is controlled with medications, how do we taper off or hopefully eliminate them? If not already implemented, we can begin one or several CAM approaches, monitor for success, and if our BP falls, we can begin to reduce our medications. That should give most of us reason to strongly consider complementary and alternative medical therapies in our efforts to control our BP. Wouldn't it be great to reduce or eliminate our need for prescription medication?

That brings us to what the AHA calls "refractory hypertension," defined as blood pressure not at goal while taking three or more medications. You'd think three medicines at standard dosages should control anyone's blood pressure, but not always. Figuring out how to help these individuals is one of our toughest challenges.

The AHA also includes under this category "multiple drug side effects," regardless of BP level. These are circumstances where we want to adjust doses or change medications in an effort to reduce side effects as much as possible, but not make reductions only to watch blood pressures rise. A two-edged sword, to be sure. At this point, we want to do everything we can to help get that person's BP as low as possible. It might never get to goal, but we want to get it as low as we can.

Here is where we would pull out all the stops—diet, lifestyle changes, and proven CAMs. With these in place, we would begin to adjust medication dosages and maybe change the class of medicine, all in an effort to control an elevated blood pressure and reduce the incidence and severity of side effects.

So there's the approach to incorporating complementary and alternative medicine into your strategy to control blood pressure. As long as you choose something that's proven to be effective, this is a reasonable and advisable plan. Make sure it fits you and your lifestyle, commit to making an effort, and give it a chance.

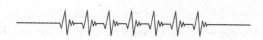

35

I've Tried Everything!

Dave Jernigan paced the tiled floor of room 2. He looked up and shook his head as I closed the door behind me. Lisa sat in the corner, smiled, and resumed her texting.

"I see you've brought reinforcements," I said, nodding to his wife.

"I wanted her here so she could confirm how hard I've been working, Doc. It's been about six weeks, and I don't think my blood pressure's where it should be."

"What makes you think that?" I leaned against the counter and opened his chart to the top page, studied his vital signs, and tossed the chart onto the exam table.

"Well, I didn't listen to you last time and made the mistake of checking my blood pressure every week or so at the drugstore. One week it would be okay, and the next it would be really high. Heck, I checked it twice one time and got two different readings. I mean *really* different."

"That's when we went online and found a good blood pressure cuff and meter," Lisa said. "Much more consistent, and *I* think more accurate."

"Still not where it needs to be." Dave shook his head again and looked at his medical record. "What did the nurse get today?"

"Well, there's good news and some…challenging news. The good thing is you've lost a couple of pounds since your last visit. That's got to be helping."

"I've been working hard at it. You can ask Lisa. I'm exercising every day and really cutting down on my carbs. I haven't had ice cream in more than—"

"How about three days," Lisa said. "You didn't think I noticed, but I did."

"Well…maybe. But no rice or potatoes, and I try to stay away from anything with sugar in it. So I *should* be losing some weight. But what about my blood pressure? What is it today?"

"That's the challenging part. It's 148 over 92. Better than last time, but not where we want it."

"And exactly where is that again?" Lisa dropped the cell phone to her lap and looked at me.

"Ideal would be 120 over 80, but our target right now is less than 140 over 90—consistently."

"That's about what I got at home this morning with our new cuff," Dave said. "I just can't seem to get it lower than that."

"He *has* been working hard on this, Dr. Lesslie. Aside from the ice cream the other night, he's really watched his diet. And he's exercising more than ever. We have a stationary bike, and he's on it for more than half an hour every day."

"And Lisa and I try to walk every evening," Dave added. "And I'm using free weights. I'm trying everything, just like you said."

"What about the salt?"

He glanced at his wife. "We took the saltshaker off the table, and Lisa doesn't use much at all with her cooking. Took some time to get used to, but after a while, it's not so bad. So yeah, we're really paying attention to that too."

I nodded and thought about how else I could advise him. It sounded like he was making the important lifestyle changes and remained motivated. That was the critical part that doesn't come in a pill or a liquid. You either are or you're not, and Dave definitely was motivated.

"I have to confess—I went online and bought some herbal stuff that's supposed to help. Green tea extract. Comes in a capsule, and I've been taking it for about a week. Nothing yet, but they claim it's supposed to help."

"What do you think about that?" Lisa glanced at Dave and then at me.

"It's worth a try," I answered. "There's some data that indicates it might help you lose weight, and that's always a good thing. But it's probably not going to fix your blood pressure."

"And there's the ginseng I ordered. Somebody at work told me it was supposed to help lower your blood pressure, but I couldn't take it. Tried to, but it made me feel funny, and I stopped."

Lisa shook her head and studied her husband. "Tell Dr. Lesslie about the vinegar."

"Vinegar?" I waited for a response, barely able to suppress a chuckle.

"Well, you see…"

"His Aunt Alice told him to take a tablespoon of vinegar three times a day, and it would purify his blood. And then his blood pressure would be normal."

"And?"

"Have you ever tried to drink vinegar straight up? I mean, it's pretty nasty. I've been doing it for three weeks now, and still can't get used to the taste."

Motivated. He had to be.

We needed to discuss putting Dave on some medication. He had worked hard at the things I recommended, and his blood pressure was still too high. And while he had expressed his willingness to be on drugs for this problem, some people ultimately resist the idea of being on medicine long term, maybe forever.

"I need some medication, Doc. It's time, don't you think?"

"He doesn't want to end up like some of the others in his family," Lisa quietly added. "What would you recommend?"

"Okay, I want you to continue with your diet, exercise, and salt restriction. But you can stop the vinegar. Let me give you a couple of ideas about medications, and we can decide what to do next."

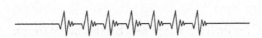

36

Pearls from the Experts

Before we get started here, just who are these experts and why do they deserve our attention? Fortunately for us, the recognition and treatment of high blood pressure has been addressed by some of the best medical minds in our country. They've come together, evaluated the latest and most compelling research studies, and put their findings in an easily accessible and understandable report. No evidence of conflict of interest here, and no obvious sources of bias. Just good, solid stuff.

This is a large group, and a complete listing of its members can be found on the website of the National Institutes of Health. The document they wrote is titled JNC 8 and is the *Eighth Report of the Joint National Committee on Prevention, Detection, Evaluation, and Treatment of High Blood Pressure.* Whew, that's a mouthful. But the title says it all. And yes, there was a seventh report, and at some point in the future there will be a ninth. In the meantime, this document gives physicians a lot of good information and direction as we help our patients control their blood pressures.

We've referred to their recommendations throughout this book, but let's take a look at some points they believed were compelling and important. If it seems a little technical, bear with me. This is the information you need to understand in order to be a partner with your healthcare provider. The more you know and the more you question, the better your results will be. This represents the latest in our thoughts about treating hypertension, though some areas remain a little controversial and will be clarified with the passage of time and completion of ongoing studies. A little more about that later, but here are some things to keep in mind.

1. In the general population, aged sixty or older, pharmacologic treatment should be started if the systolic blood pressure (SBP) is 150 or greater or the diastolic blood pressure (DBP) is 90 or greater. The goal of treatment should be a pressure of less than 150/90. This is pretty straightforward, achievable, and actually a little less intense than previous guidelines. Some controversy exists here, and as they have been in the past, these numbers are subject to change.

2. In the general population under sixty, start medication if the DBP is 90 or greater, with a goal of reducing it to under 90. See the difference here? In this age group, the management focus is on the diastolic pressure and not the systolic. A little departure from previous guidelines, but supported by solid evidence.

3. Also, for those under sixty, start medication if the SBP is equal to or greater than 140, with the goal being less than 140. The evidence is not as strong here, but it still remains a guideline.

4. In those of us older than eighteen with chronic kidney disease, the blood pressure goal needs to be less than 140/90, with the anticipation that two or more medications will most likely be required.

5. In those older than eighteen with type 1 or 2 diabetes, the blood pressure goal is also less than 140/90.

6. In the general nonblack population, including those with diabetes, initial blood pressure treatment should include a thiazide-type diuretic, calcium channel blocker, ACE inhibitor, or an angiotensin receptor blocker (ARB). This is getting a little technical, but these drugs represent the major classes of medications used for the treatment of hypertension, without listing a preferential order. We'll be looking at these later.

7. In the general black population, including those with diabetes, initial medications should include a thiazide-type diuretic or a calcium channel blocker. This is where things get a little tricky. One size doesn't fit all, and we need to pay attention to specific recommendations for specific groups of people. This advice is based on a mountain of medical research, studying what works best for some and not as well for others.

8. In those older than eighteen with chronic kidney disease, initial (or add-on) blood pressure treatment should include an ACE inhibitor or an ARB to improve kidney outcomes. This applies to all patients with chronic kidney disease (and that's a bunch of us) regardless of race or diabetes status.

9. The main objective of treatment is to reach the blood pressure goal and stay there. If the goal hasn't been reached within one month, it's time to increase the dose of the first drug, switch drugs within the same class, or add a second one. If the goal cannot be reached with two drugs at maximum recommended doses, it's time to add a third.

There are a few more points we need to keep in mind.

- In persons older than fifty years, systolic blood pressure greater than 140 mm Hg is a much more important cardiovascular disease (CVD) risk factor than diastolic blood pressure.

- The risk of CVD beginning at 115/75 *doubles* with each incremental increase of 20/10 mm Hg.

- Individuals who have a normal blood pressure at age fifty-five still have a 90 percent lifetime risk of developing hypertension.

- Most patients with hypertension will ultimately require two or more medications to achieve goal.

- If at the first diagnosis of hypertension the blood pressure is more than 20/10 above goal, strong consideration should be given to starting two drugs at the outset.

- And here's the real kicker: The most effective therapy pre-scribed by the most careful clinician will control hyperten-sion only if patients are motivated. Sometimes that's the hard part. For any treatment to work, it requires the active involve-ment of both patient and physician.

So there's a framework to keep in mind. Earlier, we mentioned the mountain of studies that supported these guidelines. The studies included tens of thousands of people—men and women of all ages, sizes, races, and locales. And they are ongoing. As soon as one area of concern is stud-ied, others quickly present themselves, needing to be defined. And the researchers doing this work seem to be quite adept at developing acro-nyms to name them. Consider the following examples:

ALLHAT—Antihypertensive and Lipid-Lowering Treat-ment to Prevent Heart Attack Trial

REIN—Ramipril (an ACE inhibitor) Efficacy in Nephrop-athy (kidney damage) study

SAVE—Survival and Ventricular Enlargement study

HOPE—Heart Outcomes Prevention Evaluation study

AASK—African American Study of Kidney Disease and Hypertension

LIFE—Losartan (an ARB) Intervention for Endpoint Reduction in Hypertension study

COPERNICUS—Carvedilol (a calcium channel blocker) Prospective Randomized Cumulative Survival Study

Wow. It seems obvious that we need simple titles to keep these stud-ies straight. I'm just glad someone is clever enough to do it, and I'm wait-ing for SAYWHAT?—the Study That Addresses All Your Worries About Hypertension And Its Treatment.

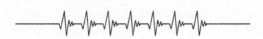

37

You Gotta Know Your Numbers

Heart Don't Fail Me Now

Shep Ballard coughed twice and sat up in bed. His breath, coming in raspy, quick catches, awakened his wife.

"What's the matter?" Diane switched on the bedside light. "It's that cough again, isn't it?"

The sixty-two-year-old was hunched over, rivulets of sweat coursing down his face and dripping onto the sheet.

"You're soaking wet." Diane pulled the bed covers away from her husband and placed a hand on his damp forehead. "I don't think you have a fever, but I don't like all this sweating. Could it be the medicine Dr. Hamilton gave you?"

Shep shook his head, struggling for breath. Between gasps he was able to mutter, "I don't know. I thought it was just an antibiotic."

Shep had seen his family physician two weeks earlier. Cough, congestion, fatigue.

"I think you've got a bad case of bronchitis," Ben Hamilton had told him. "We're seeing a lot of that going around now, and some antibiotics should clear it right up."

A prescription for a Z-pack and some cough medicine hadn't cleared it right up, and a week later, Shep was back in the office.

"I'm not getting any better, Doc. Still coughing and still tired. Especially after doing any walking. And steps—well, I find a way to avoid them whenever I can."

Hamilton glanced at Shep's medical record. No fever today, and his blood pressure...a little high at 150/102. But that was about normal for him. He continued flipping through the chart, glancing at lab reports and at an EKG done five years earlier. Shep had always been in decent health, and except for his blood pressure, had never had any serious medical problems. The only medicine he took was a fluid pill for his hypertension, and while that had never brought his pressure into the desired range, it was all Shep had wanted to try.

Hamilton's eyes came to rest over his handwritten scrawl at the bottom of one page. *White-coat syndrome.* He nodded, closed the chart, and tossed it onto the exam table.

"Let's take another listen to your chest."

The cold stethoscope pressed against Shep's back and he flinched.

"Sorry about that," Hamilton muttered. "Take a couple of deep breaths." The family practitioner listened for a few moments, and then slid the stethoscope into a lab-coat pocket. "Still got some noises going on there, and now some wheezing. How bad is your shortness of breath?"

Shep shook his head and his brow furrowed. "I guess I *have* been short of breath, but it's mainly at night, and the real problem has been this cough that won't go away. But what's this about wheezing? I don't have asthma or anything like that, do I?"

"No, don't worry about asthma." Hamilton pulled a prescription pad from another coat pocket and began scribbling. "It's all just part of this bronchitis of yours. I'm going to give you another antibiotic—something stronger this time—and put you on an inhaler to help with that wheezing."

"And cough medicine," Shep reminded him. "Something that will help me get some sleep at night. That's when I really start coughing."

Now, a week after that last doctor's visit, Shep Ballard sat in front of me on the bed of room 4 in the ER. Diane stood at his side, her eyes unable to disguise her fear.

"It's getting worse, Dr. Lesslie," Shep began between halting, labored breaths. "I can't sleep lying down anymore. I just start...smothering."

I had listened to his story and noted the half-dozen red flags popping up with each passing minute.

"Any chest pain or history of heart disease?"

"No, just the blood pressure thing," he answered, shaking his head. "And no diabetes. I've always been in good health until...this."

Diane cast a quick glance at me and then at her husband.

Shep's blood pressure was 190/110. And his heart rate was fast but regular. He still had the wheezing Dr. Hamilton had heard, and the noises he had mentioned—fine, wet sounds at the bases of both sides of his chest.

I ran two fingers over his left jugular vein, compressing the blood out of it, then releasing the pressure. It immediately filled again, bulging as it disappeared underneath his jawbone.

"What does that mean?" Diane's eyes were fixed on my fingers and her husband's neck.

"Well..." I stroked my chin and studied the man in front of me.

The diagnosis was obvious, confirmed by an EKG, chest X-ray, and cardiac ultrasound. The ultrasound bothered me most. His heart valves were fine, but his ejection fraction—a measure of the efficiency of the pumping action of his heart—was less than half of what it should have been. Shep was in heart failure and clearly on a slippery slope. He needed help, and he needed it now.

"How did this happen, Dr. Lesslie?" Diane was standing at the head of the stretcher, her hand on her husband's shoulder. "Shep has never had any heart trouble. And now heart failure? I don't understand."

"The most likely cause is his underlying high blood pressure," I said. She had told me about his constant borderline readings in Dr. Hamilton's office. "He doesn't have any other risk factors like smoking or an elevated cholesterol level. But when your heart has to constantly work hard to pump blood throughout your body, that strain can cause some damage and changes in the muscle. Eventually your heart gets tired and doesn't work as well, and finally begins to...fail."

"My blood pressure?" Shep looked up at me. "I didn't think it was anything serious—nothing dangerous. Is that what—"

Diane gently patted his shoulder. "Okay. Where do we go from here?"

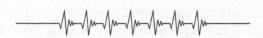

38

When It Comes to BP Medicines, What Choices Do We Have?

This area of medicine has exploded over the past ten to twenty years. We've learned a lot about the causes of high blood pressure and have been able to target specific medicines for specific problems. There are a couple of interesting points we need to keep in mind as we begin any prescription medication, and that's especially true for those used in treating our hypertension.

First, we have four main classes of drugs to choose from. Each of these is equally effective in lowering our blood pressure, with between 40 to 50 percent of us reaching goal with just one medication from any one of these four groups. There is significant variation from person-to-person in our response to a specific class of drug—or even with drugs within the same class—so choosing the right medication can take some time and patience. The bottom line is to lower our pressures, and the evidence from several large and recent studies is that it really doesn't matter which drug you use, as long as your blood pressure is controlled. We'll receive the same amount of cardio-protection once our BP goal has been met. That's good news and makes the management of this problem at little easier.

Also making it a little easier is the recently revised approach to adjusting medications. Historically, if you were started on a blood pressure medication, your physician would max out the dosage until you reached your goal. If unsuccessful, it would be time to add another drug. The problem is that most side effects increase with increasing dosages, something we'd like to avoid if at all possible. And if the second drug didn't work after its dose was maxed out, it would be time to add a third. This is called the "tiered approach," and it is no longer the recommended way to treat hypertension.

If you are on one BP drug (monotherapy) and don't reach goal in a reasonable time, the next step is to change drug classes. Try a different drug and see if it works. This can be done several times until something is successful. The additional advice now is *not* to max out the dose for each of these drugs, but to first try the half-standard dosage. It turns out that this affords most of the same BP lowering as the full dose, without many of the side effects. And remember from our discussions of measuring our pressures, the effectiveness of treatment should be assessed with home readings—or preferably an ambulatory BP monitoring—until we are at goal.

Speaking of goal, we need to keep in mind that for those of us under sixty, those numbers are anything less than 140/90. If over sixty, we'll be happy with 150/90 but would like to see it lower, as long as this can be achieved without the development of side effects.

We've talked here about monotherapy, starting out with just one medication. Is there a time when we should consider beginning with a combination of two drugs? The answer is yes. If our blood pressure is more than 20/10 mm Hg over our goal, we're probably not going to get there with one medicine only. Most experts recommend starting off with two drugs and adjusting the classes and doses accordingly.

Four Classes of BP Medicines

So what are these classes of drugs we keep talking about? As noted, we have four classes to choose from, each representing a different type of medication defined by how it attacks the problem of hypertension.

The first class is *thiazide diuretics*—the "water pills." These have been around for a while and have proven to be safe and effective. We're going to consider these and the other classes in more detail, but keep in mind that each of these classes is roughly equal in their ability to normalize an elevated blood pressure.

Next are the *calcium channel blockers,* a large group with subtle differences in how they act and some of the other positive things they do for us.

The *ACE inhibitors* are another important group of drugs that lower blood pressure as well as protect our kidneys and brains.

And the fourth class is the *angiotensin receptor blockers* (ARBs). They are sometimes lumped together with the ACE inhibitors because the two classes act on similar, related sites. But there are important differences, and we'll be considering these a little later.

If you're taking a beta-blocker (Inderal, Corgard, atenolol, metoprolol), you've probably noticed that these drugs are not listed among the four classes of BP medications we've been considering. That's because beta-blockers are no longer considered to be first-line drugs in the treatment of hypertension. We'll examine why this is so and in what circumstances they should be utilized.

Okay, with four classes to choose from—each roughly equivalent in their effectiveness—where do we start? Which one do we pick first?

The good news is that it probably doesn't matter. However, two factors should be considered before starting a specific hypertension medication—age and race. Younger individuals (up to the age of fifty) should probably be started on an ACE inhibitor. For those of us over fifty, a good choice would be a thiazide diuretic or a long-acting calcium channel blocker. Regarding race, the same choices (thiazides, calcium-channel blockers) would be indicated for African-Americans.

That's a quick overview of our blood pressure medicines. Now we need to take a closer look at each of these classes.

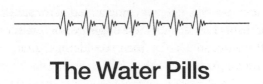

39

The Water Pills

Or to be more technically correct, the "diuretics," from the Greek word *diurosso,* meaning "I gotta go now!" Diuretics, water pills, fluid pills—they're all the same. In this chapter, we'll refer to this class of blood pressure medication as the diuretics.

For many years, these drugs were the mainstay of hypertension treatment. While they remain important and integral in the treatment of blood pressure problems, diuretics no longer reign as the "first line" drug. There is no consensus as to what that should be, if anything. We need to individualize our treatment choices depending on age, sex, race, and most importantly other medical conditions. But the diuretics have a long and well-deserved place in our arsenal of drugs.

Just how do these medications work? This is really pretty simple. These chemicals cause an increase in urine production and excretion. There are several classes of medications within this group, each producing increased urine in a different physiologic way.

The most commonly used in the treatment of hypertension are the thiazide diuretics, named after their chemical nomenclature. They exert their action at a specific location in the kidney, inhibiting the reabsorption of sodium and chloride from the urine, leading to increased water loss along with these electrolytes. There are some other as yet undefined mechanisms by which these drugs lower blood pressure, but for the most part, the "diuresis" or increased urine production is how they work. It's a subtle increase, so you're not heading for a bathroom twenty minutes after taking your pill.

That happens when you take a "loop diuretic," so named because of where it acts in your kidney—a site different from the thiazides. The most familiar drug here is Lasix, a potent diuretic used in the treatment of heart failure and certain kidney diseases. It acts quickly and produces significant urine and fluid losses. In the past, this medicine has been used illicitly by athletes, such as boxers and wrestlers, who had to make a specific weight. They would take some Lasix, visit the bathroom (frequently), and quickly drop the necessary pounds. Illegal now, of course (wink wink).

In addition to these thiazide and loop diuretics, there are several other types of drugs within this class. Some are tailored to spare potassium, and some to produce what's called an "osmotic diuresis." Mannitol is one of these, chemically related to the simple molecule glucose. It's used to draw excess fluid out of the brain in an effort to lower increased intracranial pressure resulting from a stroke or head trauma. And speaking of glucose—simple blood sugar—this is another potent "osmotic diuretic." When increased, as in an undiagnosed or undertreated diabetic, it is excreted in our urine, where it draws water along with it. That's why diabetics with elevated blood sugars experience increased urination, thirst, and ultimately a dangerous weight loss.

But back to our thiazide diuretics. This is the group most commonly used in our fight against hypertension. If you're being treated for high blood pressure, you're probably taking one of these right now, most likely hydrochlorothiazide (HCTZ) either by itself or in combination with another drug. This is the most frequently used thiazide and has been a mainstay for many years. That may be changing, and we'll consider why in our next chapter.

Another thiazide that's been around for a while is chlorthalidone. It's not used as much as HCTZ, but that's changing. More about that as well. It's available as a generic, making it cheaper, yet it's very effective—both good things. Other trade names containing the thiazides are listed below, and you might be able to find your medication listed here.

Lotensin HCT—an ACE inhibitor with HCTZ
Vaseretic—another ACE with HCTZ
Monopril—ACE plus HCTZ

Micardis HCT—an ARB with HCTZ
Benicar HCT—another ARB with HCTZ
Lopressor HCT—a beta blocker with HCTZ
Tenoretic—A beta blocker with chlorthalidone
Aldoril—an old medicine with HCTZ
Hydropres—a *really* old medicine with HCTZ
Maxzide—a different type of diuretic with HCTZ (a double whammy)

This is only a partial list, but it gives us an idea of the types of drugs we're talking about here. The thiazide diuretics are an important part of managing hypertension—either alone or in combination.

But how do you choose which one is best for you? How do we make sense of the ever-multiplying choices of medications? We're going to tackle that question next.

40

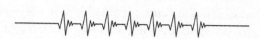

Diuretics: The Pros and Cons

Remember that most antihypertensive medications by themselves are able to satisfactorily lower blood pressure in 30 to 50 percent of people taking them. That's not everyone, but it's a lot of us. This is true for diuretics as well, and a lot of us might be taking only hydrochlorothiazide (HCTZ) or (preferably) chlorthalidone and have well-controlled pressures.

That's one of the pros. Another big benefit is their cost. These are inexpensive medications, costing just a few dollars for a month's supply. And they have few interactions with other medications. Almost all of us can take them without having any problems. In addition to hypertension, they are used effectively either alone or with other medications to treat heart failure, polycystic ovary disease, and some types of kidney stones.

But the biggest plus for diuretics is that they work. In fact, the thiazide-type diuretics have been the cornerstone of high blood pressure treatment in most clinical trials, and they've led the other classes of medications when it comes to preventing complications like heart attacks and strokes.

There are a few cons though. As with all of the antihypertensive medications, those taking them can experience episodes of low blood pressure, sometimes resulting in dangerous falls. This is not as frequent as with other types of drugs, but it does happen. Dehydration can occur as well—understandable since these are "fluid pills."

Specific problems with thiazide diuretics can include low levels of potassium (lost through increased urine production), which can sometimes be serious. This can be prevented with increased potassium intake through potassium-rich foods, such as cantaloupes, raisins, bananas, prunes, yogurt, and flounder. Salt substitutes, such as Lite Salt—half potassium and half sodium—are also an easy and effective way to increase your dietary potassium.

These diuretics can also cause increases in uric acid—the naturally occurring chemical responsible for gout—and low levels of magnesium, sometimes resulting in muscle cramps and weakness. Importantly, thiazides can increase lipid levels and interfere with how the body handles glucose, making control of diabetes more difficult. Most people don't experience these problems, but they are out there. The key, as with all medications, is to use the lowest dose possible.

Something else to be aware of is the emerging issue of which thiazide diuretic we physicians should be prescribing for our patients. In the past, this was simple. For many years, HCTZ has been the most commonly used diuretic, prescribed either by itself or in combination with a host of other antihypertensive medicines, noted in the previous chapter. New information is calling this into question and changing the recommendations here. Let's take a look.

HCTZ, while effective in lowering blood pressure, is relatively short-acting, exerting its effects for only six to twelve hours. This can make it difficult to accurately monitor your blood pressure depending on when you take the medicine. Many of our patients take their blood pressure medicine in the morning, within hours of an appointment in our clinic. The HCTZ will be working at that point, and their blood pressure might be fine. But what happens later in the day or during the night? And what happens if, as do many of our patients, they come to their appointment having fasted and haven't taken any of their medications? That's a big question and concern.

But here's something interesting and important. Remember all those acronyms for research studies? One of them, ALLHAT, presented some fascinating findings. The Antihypertensive and Lipid-Lowering Treatment to Prevent Heart Attack Trial followed more than forty-one thousand people with high blood pressure and assigned them to several single medication regimens. These included amlodipine (a calcium channel blocker), lisinopril (an ACE inhibitor), doxazocin (an alpha-blocker, stopped prematurely after an increased incidence of heart failure was observed in those taking it), and chlorthalidone (an older thiazide diuretic). After the doxazocin was discontinued, the three remaining drugs all lowered blood pressures as well as the incidence of coronary heart disease and heart attacks. But people taking chlorthalidone (we'll refer to it as CTD) had a significantly reduced risk of heart failure and of several important cardiovascular diseases. A lowly fluid pill? And more so than HCTZ? That's right. So what do we know about this drug? A lot, and it's impressive stuff.

First, this medication has been around for quite a while, initially marketed as Hygroton. I'm not sure how or why it fell into relative disuse, but HCTZ has eclipsed it at this point in time. Puzzling, since CTD is 1.5 to 2 times as potent as HCTZ. This is significant since we want to use the smallest amount of medication possible. And it stays in your system longer than HCTZ (twenty-four to seventy-two hours versus six to twelve). When compared to HCTZ, CTD significantly reduces the risk of cardiovascular events and lowers systolic blood pressure better and longer than HCTZ. As with HCTZ, we need to keep an eye on our potassium level, but this can easily be managed.

All of this sounds great, so why aren't more of us taking it instead of HCTZ? That's a good question, and one that a growing number of blood pressure experts are addressing. Current recommendations are that CTD should now be the *thiazide diuretic of choice*, begun at a dose of 12.5 to 25 mgs. One possible exception would be among frail older persons whose blood pressure is less than 10 mm Hgs above goal. Low-dose HCTZ might still be a good choice here.

So if you're taking HCTZ, either alone or in combination, what should you do? How do you approach this with your healthcare provider? I can tell you what we're doing in our practice. At each office visit, we're making every effort to switch our patients on HCTZ to CTD. It can be done, even with those of us on multiple medications and combination drugs. And if you want to do this but meet resistance? Ask your physician if they've reviewed the ALLHAT data. That should elicit an interesting response.

The points here are simple. Thiazide diuretics are effective drugs for the treatment of hypertension. We need to be aware of the possible side effects and complications and do what we can to prevent them. And our thiazide of choice needs to be chlorthalidone.

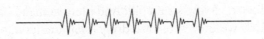

41

The Calcium Channel Blockers (CCBs)

Before we take a look at this class of medications, let's see exactly what we're talking about. Here is a list of the most frequently used; you might recognize one of your medications in this group There are two types of calcium channel blockers (CBC), and we'll refer to them simply as I and II (arbitrary but adequate for this discussion). It's an important distinction because of their respective actions and side effects.

Type I
Diltiazem (Cardizem, Tiazac, Dilacor)
Verapamil (Calan, Isoptin, Covera)
Type II
Amlodipine (Norvasc)
Felodipine (Plendil)
Nicardipine (Cardene)
Nifedipine (Adalat, Procardia)

These drugs are prescribed individually or in combination with several of the other classes of high blood pressure medicines.

Let's start with the basics: exactly what is a *calcium channel* and why would we want to block it? The best way to think of this is that these channels represent a pathway within cell walls that allow for the movement of specific electrolytes (in this setting referred to as *ions*). These might be sodium or potassium or, in this instance, calcium. This movement of ions results in energy exchange, electrical impulses, transfer of chemical charges—a bunch of stuff. All of these are naturally occurring and needed cellular actions within our bodies.

The movement of calcium through specific *channels* is one of those, and if we can block that movement, we can stop the resulting actions. This might be slowing the conduction of other electrical impulses through the heart, or decreasing the force of contraction of cardiac muscle fibers, or causing blood vessels to relax and dilate. In the right setting, all of these actions might be useful.

This class of medication was discovered by a German researcher in 1964, and the first available drug was verapamil. This new class represented a big step forward in the treatment of high blood pressure and other cardiac diseases. It wasn't long before others were developed, with specific tweaks leading to the development of the type I and type II categories.

The CCBs are used not only in the treatment of high blood pressure, but also for angina and to slow the heart rate when this becomes necessary. In addition to these actions, they can also help relieve cerebral vasospasm (an important and beneficial action in the brain of someone who has suffered a ruptured aneurysm and whose surrounding blood vessels have squeezed shut), and with Raynaud's disease, another type of vasospasm.

We mentioned that these drugs block our calcium channels. This action results in four important outcomes:

- By acting on the muscles of the heart, the force of contraction is reduced.

- By acting on the muscle tissue in our blood vessels, they reduce the contraction of our arteries, causing them to relax and resulting in a larger internal diameter—something important called *vasodilation.*

- By slowing down the electrical conduction in our heart, they can slow down the heart rate.

- By blocking chemical pathways in our adrenal glands—those leading to the production of hormones that can elevate our blood pressure—they can *lower* our blood pressure.

For those interested in a little more technical information (keeping in mind that most *physicians* don't keep this stuff straight), these four mechanisms are what separates the CCBs into those two main classes we listed earlier. One group exerts its action mainly by causing vasodilation, thus lowering the blood pressure. The other class affects the cells of the heart by causing less forceful contraction and a slower heart rate. And then there are some newer drugs that combine a little of both.

These different mechanisms have to be kept in mind when we give them to someone with high blood pressure. For instance, if someone has mild or moderate heart failure, certain CCBs can cause further weakening of the heart and throw them into life-threatening failure. So while these are potent and effective medications for hypertension and other serious medical problems, they are also potentially dangerous. And unlike some other types of blood pressure medications, CCBs, while very effective in lowering blood pressure, have not *yet* been proven to reduce the incidence of death caused by cardiovascular disease.

In the next chapter, we'll look at some of the other important benefits of the CCBs as well as their side effects.

42

CCBs: The Pros and Cons

The calcium channel blockers (CCBs) are important weapons in our fight against hypertension. They are powerful medications capable of significantly lowering blood pressure and, when necessary, slowing a rapid heart rate. They are usually not used alone but in combination with other classes of medications, frequently an ACE inhibitor (such as Lotrel and Tarka). Another advantage is that they've been on the market for a while and their cost has fallen, though they're not as inexpensive as hydrochlorothiazide (HCTZ). But then, nothing is.

CCBs are effective in the prevention of migraine headaches and are capable of helping with this debilitating problem when other therapies aren't. And I mentioned Raynaud's disease. This is something a lot of us have to deal with, myself included. When our hands are exposed to the cold, one or more of our fingers blanch and sometimes become painful. While not usually indicative of any serious vascular problem, it can be a nuisance as well as a cause for questions from your grandchildren. "Papa, why are your fingertips so white?" The CCBs can help with this, due to their ability to cause vasodilation. This counters the vasospasm that causes the lack of blood flow. Something to think about if you have this problem and it has begun to bother you.

We mentioned the use of CCBs in patients with chest pain (angina) and fast or irregular heartbeats, and it's also one of the few treatments available for *pulmonary hypertension,* another debilitating disease caused by thickening and spasm of the arteries in our lungs.

So the CCBs are effective and helpful drugs, but they also have some bothersome and serious side effects. Before we talk about those, this class of blood pressure medication has been given a bad rap in the press—undeserved and deserving of being debunked.

The first has to do with an alleged increase in heart attacks in people taking these medicines. This story hit the news a little more than ten years ago, persisted, and was finally determined to be unfounded.

Then there was the disquieting claim that CCBs were associated with an increased risk of cancer, particularly of the breast. Again, no causal link has ever been established between these drugs and the development of any type of cancer.

And finally, there have been reports of an increased incidence of gastrointestinal bleeding in elderly individuals taking these medicines. Again not true.

Why bring these things to your attention? First, you might be taking one of these drugs, read these reports, and become worried unnecessarily. And second, these demonstrate the willingness of our media to inform us of dramatic "new findings," even when they have no basis in fact. That steams me.

But there are some potential problems associated with the use of the CCBs. Some of these are *minor* problems ("minor" being open to interpretation and frequently defined by whether it affects you or someone else), such as constipation, flushing, nausea, fatigue, swelling in the feet and lower legs, and sometimes various rashes. These side effects are usually dose-related, meaning the higher the dose you take, the greater the chance of developing the side effect. And most are self-limiting—they begin early after you start the medicine and frequently disappear after a short period of time (usually days or a few weeks).

There are real and more serious side effects with these medicines, and they relate to their mechanisms. Because of their ability to slow the heart rate, this side effect can result in decreased blood getting to the brain, causing dizziness and sometimes near-syncope—almost blacking out. Subsequent falls can result in fractures of the wrists, hips, and spine.

And since the CCBs cause vasodilation, the same problems can occur. Excessive pooling of blood in our vascular system can result in markedly low blood pressure, dizziness, and again those dangerous falls.

These are powerful drugs, capable of great help and great harm. That fact was brought home to me one afternoon in the ER. A thirty-year-old woman, we'll call her Ellie, was brought to the hospital in the backseat of her friend's SUV. The blaring horn just outside the ambulance entrance got our attention, and we rushed out to find her slumped over, unresponsive, and barely breathing. Her friend was less than helpful, simply telling us that she "hadn't been acting right" for a couple of hours.

Once in the ER, we took her straight to the cardiac room, started two IVs, and hooked her to the cardiac monitor. The usual measures in this circumstance didn't help and didn't give us any guidance. Her blood sugar was normal, BP was fine, heart rate in the 80s and regular, no needle tracks on her arms or legs, and there was no evidence of any trauma. Her friend, once again, had nothing to say.

We continued to work with Ellie, checking labs and a portable chest X-ray, searching for a cause of her unresponsiveness. And then her heart started slowing down. When she came into the department, it was in the low 80s and her blood pressure was 100/60. Nothing unusual for a slender young woman. But in front of our eyes, the blipping of the cardiac monitor slowed—into the 70s, then the 60s. And her blood pressure started to fall as well.

I confronted her friend once more, asking her for any information she might have. Nothing. Ellie had no medical problems and didn't use drugs or alcohol. Her friend had no useful information. But something bothered me—she wouldn't look me in the eyes.

Heart rate in the 50s now and blood pressure 60 over something.

"Listen, we're going to lose Ellie. If you know something that could help and don't tell me, you'll have to live with that."

Finally, she told me that Ellie had just broken off a long relationship, was upset and depressed, and had taken some of her father's medication. Not a lot, but it seemed to have been enough to make her sleepy, and then unresponsive.

"What type of medicine was it?"

The friend wasn't sure but thought it might be something "for high blood pressure."

Slowing heart rate, falling blood pressure. This fit the picture of an overdose of a calcium channel blocker. Not something we typically see with intentional overdoses, but this had to be it.

The antidote for this poisoning is IV calcium and lots of it. We needed to overcome the excessive blockade and reverse the action of whatever calcium channel blocker Ellie had taken.

We pushed fluids, pushed the calcium, and pushed other drugs to raise her blood pressure.

And we lost her.

These are potent drugs. Usually very safe and very helpful. But as with all medications, they have to be handled with care.

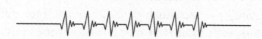

43

The Beta-Blockers:
What They Are and How They Work

The beta-blockers (ß-blockers) were some of the first significant medicines used in our battle against heart disease. In 1964, an English scientist developed the first clinically useful drug in this class—propranolol. It radically changed how we were able to treat angina, and later it was used in the treatment of high blood pressure.

They are called beta-blockers because they block the beta-receptors located on many cell walls throughout our body. We're in the realm of physiology now, but bear with me, this is important.

So we have these beta-receptors—specialized areas located on various structures that when activated, cause several important things to happen. The main *activator* is epinephrine (adrenaline), our old friend that instigates the fight-or-flight reaction. These beta-receptors are found on cells in the heart muscles, airways, arteries, kidneys, and several other areas. When adrenaline is released, it seeks out these receptors, activates them, and we see an immediate increase in our heart rates, in the strength of contraction of our heart muscles, and an opening-up of our airways—everything we need to fight or take flight.

If this action is blocked, we see the opposite reaction. Our pulse rate drops, our hearts don't beat as hard, and we don't see the bronchodilation in our lungs. That's what the beta-blockers do—they block these actions and slow everything down. That turns out to be a good thing if you have angina and are not getting as much blood flow and oxygen to your heart as needed. These medications slow down the heart and reduce the demand placed upon it. It's because of this that the use of beta-blockers in the setting of an acute heart attack has been proven to save lives. Important stuff.

Without going into too much detail, there are three different types of beta-receptors, each located in specific areas of the body. If the beta-blocker drug hits all of these willy-nilly, it falls into the nonselective category. And if it targets just one of these areas, it is selective. The earlier beta-blockers were nonselective, but as we have learned more about all of this, later generations of beta-blockers are now more selective—targeted to specific areas for specific actions. And in case you were wondering, there *are* alpha-receptors and their associated alpha-blockers. That's another class of BP medicines we'll look at later.

When it comes to managing blood pressure, beta-blockers are effective but less optimal than the other main classes of agents. As we discussed earlier, they are no longer considered a first-line choice in treating hypertension, due to the recognized increased risk of stroke and cardiac problems. Some of the later, more selective beta-blockers are safer, but are now considered an add-on-drug. However, these drugs continue to be very important in the management of a whole host of significant medical problems, including angina, atrial fibrillation, mitral valve prolapse, migraine headaches, congestive heart failure, heart attacks, various cardiac arrhythmias, and tremors.

If you're taking one of these medications and wonder where they fit in this selective/nonselective classification, here's some information:

Nonselective agents
Carvedilol
Labetalol
Nadolol
Pindolol
Sotalol

Selective agents
Atenolol
Bisoprolol
Metoprolol

Your physician had a reason for placing you on one of these medications, and if you have any questions about their use, this would be something good to discuss with him or her.

One last point about the beta-blockers, and something I find very interesting. If you play a musical instrument or engage in a competitive sport (especially something individual like golf, target shooting, or platform diving), you might have experienced "performance anxiety." Sweaty palms, rapid breathing, flushed face, trembling hands. I know *I've* been there, and it's not fun. Beta-blockers do a great job reducing this anxiety and slowing everything down. Apparently pro golfers are very familiar with its use, as are athletes who have participated in various Olympic Games. In fact, the International Olympic Committee has banned their use, attesting to their effectiveness, and hence the conferring of an unfair advantage. In this short-term and limited use, the beta-blockers have generally been very safe. That's not always the case, as we will see in the next chapter.

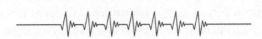

44

Beta-Blockers: The Pros and Cons

We mentioned in the last chapter that the beta-blockers are powerful drugs and very effective in the treatment of many significant diseases. When it comes to the management of hypertension, they are no longer a first-line choice and have some major drawbacks. However, there are a couple of circumstances where these drugs should be considered in the treatment of high blood pressure. The first is after an acute heart attack, and the second would be in stable patients with certain types of heart failure. In these settings, they have been proven to save lives.

There are also some major side effects of these drugs that we have to keep in mind.

The management of *heart failure* is complicated. Despite the importance of beta-blockers in the long-term treatment of this problem, these medications can sometimes worsen heart failure. It's easy to imagine how this might happen, since the action of the drug is to slow down the heart and decrease its workload. It's a delicate balance and needs to be managed by experts.

Since beta-blockers are very effective in slowing the heart rate, this action of these drugs can sometimes be excessive, producing dizziness, lightheadedness, and even loss of consciousness—all due to a reduced cardiac output and low blood pressure. This usually happens in an individual with an underlying electrical conduction problem in the heart and can be prevented by routine and simple testing.

There is a significant concern when it comes to stopping a beta-blocker, whether intentionally by your physician or by accident, such as leaving your medicine at home when you go on vacation. Sudden withdrawal of a beta-blocker can cause angina and possibly precipitate a heart attack. This usually happens when heart disease is already present, but it can occur even when there is no previous history of any coronary artery disease. Pretty scary. If the decision is made to stop your beta-blocker, you'll need to develop a tapering strategy. This will be determined by whether the medication is short-acting (propranolol, metoprolol, carvedilol) or long-acting (atenolol, long-acting metoprolol, nadolol). It makes a difference, and your physician can guide you through this process.

There are other bothersome beta-blocker side effects not related to cardiac issues. We mentioned that there are beta-receptors in the airways of our lungs, whose activation dilates our bronchioles and other smaller air passages. Beta-blockers prevent this dilation, and in the setting of significant asthma and other airway diseases, can cause bronchospasm and worsening shortness of breath. Because of this, beta-blockers should be used with caution in those of us with asthma, and then only with the selective medications and in those with only mild or moderate lung disease. Another delicate balancing act.

These drugs should also be used with caution in those of us with peripheral vascular disease, since they can potentially worsen the already reduced blood flow to our extremities. They can also complicate the management of blood-sugar levels in those of us with diabetes, and elevate potassium levels to potentially dangerous levels in those with heart failure and significant kidney disease.

Lastly, some of us will experience depression, fatigue, and sexual dysfunction while taking these medications. Not too long ago, these were felt to occur frequently with the beta-blockers. It turns out the incidence of these is much less than previously thought, yet it's something to keep in mind.

So that's about it. The bottom line here is to be aware of the potential side effects of these drugs, talk with your physician about them, and make an informed decision before you begin taking them. When used in the right circumstances and properly monitored, they can be safe and very effective at what they do.

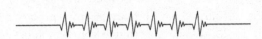

45

Keep an ACE Up Your Sleeve: The ACE Inhibitors

This class of blood pressure medicine has been in use for a while, with captopril being introduced in 1975. Since then, several other important ACE inhibitors have been developed, making this group a mainstay in the treatment of hypertension. But what exactly is an ACE? And why do we want to inhibit it?

Before captopril, investigators from around the world were discovering and exploring something called the renin-angiotensin system (RAS) and how it was central in the control of our blood volumes and blood pressures. This is going to be a little more physiology, but it's necessary, so don't turn the page. With a small amount of effort, we'll see how this all comes together, makes sense, and can be put to good use. And we'll see another clear example of how our bodies are "fearfully and wonderfully made" (Psalm 139), and how nothing has been left to chance.

I've stated earlier that I'm a visual learner. You might be as well. I like to see things, see how they flow and fit together. When I can see how that happens, I'm able to understand and remember what I'm studying. So since I'm a visual learner, I've included a diagram or flowchart of the RAS. Let's take a look. (If you or someone you care about takes an ACE inhibitor—lisinopril, ramipril, Accupril, anything ending in a "pril"—you'll want to understand this.)

Renin-Angiotensin System (RAS)

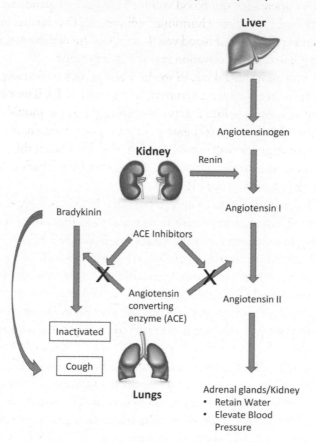

Diagram 1 by Jeff Lesslie

We'll start with our liver. This organ produces a chemical called angiotensinogen. Renin, a protein made in our kidneys, acts on angiotensinogen, converting it to another protein, angiotensin I. Okay so far? Good. Then we have specialized cells in our lungs that produce something called angiotensin converting enzyme (ACE). This is going to interact with angiotensin I and convert it into angiotensin II. This chemical is where it all seems to happen. We have angiotensin II receptors scattered throughout our bodies, and when they're activated, a lot of different things start to happen. Our heart rate goes up, the kidneys reabsorb sodium and other electrolytes (increasing our blood volume), the adrenal glands are poked and instructed to produce a hormone (aldosterone) that further increases our sodium levels, and our blood vessels constrict. All of these actions lead to…you guessed it—an elevation in our blood pressure.

Now you know how the RAS works. Let's go back to that step where our lungs produce angiotensin converting enzyme (ACE). If we can block or inhibit this ACE before it acts on angiotensin I, we should be able to stop the effects of everything else occurring downstream. And that's exactly what happens with our ACE inhibitors. They block this step, preventing those actions that elevate our blood pressures. That's how these drugs work in lowering our BP.

You'll also notice something on the chart that deals with the bradykinin system, which is important in several critical functions. There's an interesting interplay here between this system and the RAS. We can see that the bradykinins are inactivated by the angiotensin converting enzyme, and when this is blocked by our ACE inhibitors, there's a buildup of the active form of the bradykinins.

A couple of important processes occur when this happens. First, the bradykinins produce the potent chemical nitric oxide, a vasodilator that leads to a lower blood pressure. Nitric oxide is also essential when it comes to the health of our blood vessels and heart. One of the side effects of too much nitric oxide is thought to be some airway irritation and development of a nagging cough. Keep this in mind—we'll be discussing it later.

So we have our ACE inhibitors and we know where they act in this RAS. Now, how do we put them to the best use?

In addition to effectively lowering an elevated blood pressure, the ACE inhibitors have been found to be very useful in the treatment of an acute heart attack and in certain types of heart failure. We also know they are protective of our kidneys and have an important part to play in the treatment of the renal complications associated with diabetes.

These are important drugs, but our main interest here is in their use in fighting hypertension. How do they stack up against other classes of blood pressure medicines, and how do they stack up against each other?

It's important to state once more that any of the four main classes of BP medications have the potential of normalizing an elevated pressure in 40 to 50 percent of us. One class is no better than another (unless there is the presence of a few well-defined circumstances where one class might be superior or where one class should not be used at all). And we now know that the cardiovascular benefits we receive from the blood pressure medications is based on the *amount* of blood pressure lowering, not the *type* of drug being used. The critical point is to get your blood pressure to where it should be. That's what matters.

"But why did my doctor recommend an ACE inhibitor when she found out my blood pressure was 150 over 92? She said it was a good place to start."

She's right, and you've got a good doctor. With a blood pressure in this range, you'll need to get it down, and an ACE inhibitor is a good first choice. They are efficient in lowering blood pressure, and they do so with few significant side effects. And one of the long-acting drugs will give you protection throughout the day and night.

So the good news is most of us can take these drugs and get our pressures down. A few of us will have problems with them, and we'll take a look at that next.

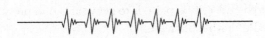

46

ACE Inhibitors: The Pros and Cons

We know that the ACE inhibitors are effective blood pressure medicines, capable of reducing our pressures by as much as 15/8 mm Hg—all by themselves. And we know they are helpful in the treatment of heart failure, medical management after a heart attack, and in the treatment of diabetic-related kidney problems. That's the good news, the pros. Now, about the cons and potential problems.

Low Blood Pressure

"I thought that was what we were trying to do?"

It is, but if our pressures get *too* low we can experience dizziness, fatigue, and even black-out spells. Falls can lead to broken bones and other significant problems we want to avoid. This can usually be prevented by starting with small doses and titrating upward gradually and carefully. Paying attention to our hydration is also very important. Most of us don't drink enough water, and if we're dehydrated, any of the blood pressure medicines can cause a dangerous fall in our BP.

Kidney Problems

"But I thought the ACE inhibitors protect the kidneys, not damage them."

Correct again, but these drugs can initially cause a slight reduction in the normal functioning of our kidneys, usually in the setting of specific types of problems and diseases such as diabetes and mild heart failure.

Any such changes are usually short-lived, but will need to be monitored. Your physician should be aware of any of the conditions that might put you at risk.

Elevated Potassium Levels

This is a common problem with our thiazide diuretics, but it can also occur with the ACE inhibitors. It has to do with the RAS system we looked at, and with the adrenal hormone aldosterone. When this part of the system is blocked, our potassium levels can rise, but unless there is significant underlying kidney disease, this will not result in a dangerous elevation. Again, your physician should be aware of the things that might make this worse and will need to monitor your potassium levels.

Cough

This turns out to be an all-too-common problem with our patients who take one of the ACE inhibitors. You might have experienced this yourself and had to change classes of medications. It affects as many as 20 percent of people treated with these drugs and can be very bothersome. It's not a serious or life-threatening problem, but it is aggravating. Here's what we know about it:

- The cough usually starts within one or two weeks after beginning the ACE inhibitor, but sometimes won't appear for as long as six months.
- All of the ACE inhibitors seem equally capable of causing this side effect.
- More women than men will develop the cough.
- Having a history of respiratory problems (asthma, chronic bronchitis) does not increase the frequency of this occurring. The cough can happen with anybody.
- It will usually go away within three or four days after stopping the ACE inhibitor, though it might take up to a month.

So what causes this cough? If we remember the RAS discussed in the last chapter and look back at diagram 1, we'll see the bradykinin sequence. When we take an ACE inhibitor, it blocks the angiotensin II pathway (lowering our blood pressure) and it also blocks the breakdown of brady-kinin. When this chemical builds up, the current thought is that it can cause irritation in our airways, and hence the cough. Be on the lookout for this if you begin taking an ACE inhibitor. The cough may be subtle yet disturb your sleep or interfere with your daily routines. And there's no effective treatment other than stopping the medicine.

Full-Blown Allergic Reactions

"Doc, my lips are all swollen and I feel funny. What's going on?"

Hmm. No insect stings. No strawberries or pineapple for breakfast. How about an ACE inhibitor? Though rare, these drugs can cause an allergic reaction—swelling of the lips, face, and tongue—that can range in symptoms from being a cosmetic nuisance to a life-threatening event. The cause is felt to be those elevated bradykinin levels again. Once this happens, the medication must be stopped immediately and never resumed. Again, this is a rare occurrence, but if you're on any of these medicines, it's something to be aware of.

Fetal Problems

If you're pregnant, possibly pregnant, or at risk of becoming pregnant, the ACE inhibitors *must* be avoided. Unlike many medications that can cause fetal problems if taken during the first trimester of pregnancy (when our organs are being formed), when taken during *any* trimester the ACE inhibitors can cause stillbirths, malformations, and deaths shortly after birth. That's scary and has to be kept in mind. How common is this? Some experts believe that about half of all newborns exposed to these drugs will have some bad effect.

So there are your pros and cons with the ACE inhibitors. On balance, the benefits far outweigh the harms, but there are a couple of things to keep in mind. Be on the lookout for the cough. Stop the medicine if you experience any swelling of the face, lips, or tongue. And avoid these if there's a chance you're pregnant or might become so.

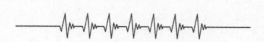

47

The Angiotensin Receptor Blockers (ARBs): Just Another ACE?

It seems that a lot of us—physicians included—sometimes confuse ACE inhibitors with the angiotensin receptor blockers (ARBs). It's easy to do, since both classes of these hypertensive drugs exert their influence within the renin-angiotensin system (RAS). But while similar, they have different actions and different side effects.

In the last couple of chapters, we looked at the ACE inhibitors and how they were able to lower blood pressure. It's important to keep the RAS diagram in mind and remember where these drugs act—inhibiting the *formation* of angiotensin II. The ARBs operate further downstream by blocking the many *actions* of angiotensin II. This chemical is a potent vasoconstrictor and is very effective at elevating our blood pressures. If we can block this action, we can lower our BP. That's how these drugs work. Diagram 2 demonstrates where this happens.

You'll also note that unlike the ACE inhibitors, the ARBs do *not* interfere with the action of angiotensin converting enzyme on the breakdown of bradykinin. This will be important when we talk about side effects.

Renin-Angiotensin System (RAS)

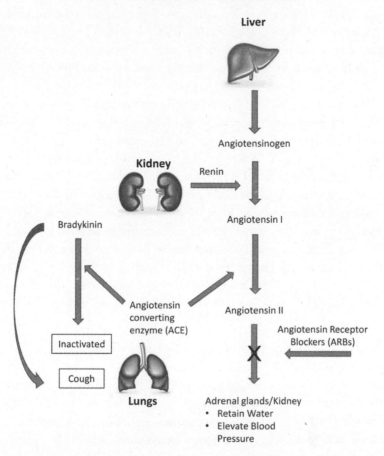

Diagram 2 by Jeff Lesslie

Just how did we discover these drugs? Well, like most pharmaceutical discoveries and innovations, this is an interesting story. In the late eighteen hundreds, a couple of scientists were experimenting with rabbits, and for some reason injecting them with kidney extracts (don't tell PETA!). They noted an increase in blood pressure in these bunnies, and eventually discovered the protein renin. Decades later, other scientists isolated additional enzymes, named angiotensin I and II, determining that these were the agents responsible for the rise in blood pressure as well as damage to the kidneys and heart. It only took filling in the blanks to figure out the RAS system. Once that was done, the move was on to find and develop drugs that would be able to block the actions of some of these enzymes, and in 1995, losartan was approved in this country as the first ARB. Others have followed, with differing potencies, benefits, and side effects.

Initially the ARBs were used primarily for the treatment of hypertension, and then only when a patient couldn't take one of the ACE inhibitors (cough or swelling of the face). It quickly became obvious that these drugs were important in their own right, and soon became one of the mainstays in the treatment of high blood pressure. As we've noted, the ARBs are now one of the four main classes used to manage hypertension.

What are some of these drugs, and how do they compare with each other? There are some differences in potency, but these are equalized by adjusting dosages. Remember—the benefit from a drug in reducing the risk of cardiovascular disease lies not with the drug itself but by its ability to lower your BP to a normal range. With that said, here's a list of some of the ARB drugs, along with their trade names. We'll divide these into groups based on how long they stay in our systems.

Relatively short acting—6-9 hours
Losartan (Cozaar)
Candesartan (Atacand)
Valsartan (Diovan)
Eprosartan (Teveten)
Longer acting—9-16 hours
Irbesartan (Avapro)
Olmesartan (Benicar)
Azilsartan (Edarbi)
The longest acting—24 hours
Telmisartan (Micardis)

This "time" business turns out to be important, since we want to be sure our blood pressure stays in the normal range all day long, without any dangerous spikes.

In addition to being effective blood pressure medicines, the ARBs are also important in the treatment of heart failure. And like the ACE inhibitors, they are protective of our kidneys, especially in those of us with diabetes.

Now, here are some interesting potential benefits of these drugs. At least one study demonstrated that losartan (Cozaar) improved sexual dysfunction in those males who needed to be treated for their hypertension. Other studies have shown that several of the ARBs (valsartan, candesartan, and telmisartan) are capable of improving this dysfunction when caused by other classes of hypertension medications. This is an important topic, at least in our clinic. Maybe in your home.

Another fascinating association has been found between the incidence and progression of Alzheimer's disease and the use of the ARBs. Those taking these drugs have less risk of developing this problem. This is still being studied, but it would be a significant development if found to be true.

And then there's the AGTR-1 gene. This affects the actions of angiotensin II at various sites in our body, and in mice at least, when this gene is partially deactivated or down-regulated, the mice live longer—as much as 25 percent longer. The ARBs appear to cause this down-regulation. While this increase in longevity would be good for our mice, it would be great for us. Interesting stuff, and something to watch for in the future.

So the ARBs are effective blood pressure medicines, and they have significant potential in other areas. Remember though—they're not "just another ACE inhibitor."

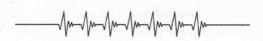

48

The ARBs: The Pros and Cons

We know the benefits of the angiotensin receptor blockers. They are very effective in lowering blood pressure, allowing about 50 percent of us to achieve our BP goal with one of these medicines just by itself. And we know it's an important drug in the treatment of heart failure and in preventing damage to the kidneys caused by diabetes. Even though these medicines are well tolerated, we need to be aware of the potential side effects that can sometimes occur.

Common adverse drug reactions can include dizziness, headaches, and an elevated potassium level. The dizziness and headaches usually resolve a week or so after starting one of these medicines, while paying attention to your potassium level is something that will need to be done as long as you're taking it. Some people have this problem more than others, and we're not sure why. So just know your levels.

If you go online (an established and significant health hazard) and look up these or any drugs, you'll find a whole host of possible adverse reactions. Most of them are usually very uncommon, and the majority will improve with the passage of a little time.

There are a few things we need to keep in mind while we're taking one of the drugs in this class. The routine procedure when someone develops a dry cough while on an ACE inhibitor is to switch them to an ARB. This almost always works, getting rid of the cough and keeping the blood pressure where it needs to be. In some instances an individual will develop the cough while on an ARB. This occurs much less frequently than with an ACE inhibitor and the treatment is the same—you'll need to stop the medicine.

This decreased incidence of cough with the ARBs makes sense. Flip back to the last chapter and take a look at diagram 2. You'll see that the bradykinin system is unaffected by the ARBs. Their action occurs downstream. This differentiates them from the ACE inhibitors and explains the cough issue. We also see less facial swelling and allergic reactions with the ARBs compared to the ACE inhibitors. Again it has to do with the bradykinin business and this makes sense once more.

The ARBs *can* produce facial swelling, though not as often as the ACE inhibitors. And while we calmly switch from an ACE inhibitor to an ARB after the development of a cough, most experts would not switch from an ACE to an ARB after a significant allergic reaction, including facial swelling. Starting one of these medicines again can sometimes be fatal. This is another example of where you *really* need to know your medications.

Similar to the ACE inhibitors, the ARBs can cause some kidney problems—again, in those individuals who are at risk for this. And they can cause some light-headedness and low blood pressure.

As with the ACE inhibitors, the ARBs *must* be avoided by women who are pregnant or who are planning to become so. In fact, if there's *any* chance of becoming pregnant, these two classes of hypertensive medications should not be used.

From time to time, we will see someone in the office who has somehow ended up on both an ACE inhibitor and an ARB. They probably received these from different physicians at different times and in different places—a real risk for "poly-pharmacy." When this happens, one of the drugs needs to be immediately stopped. Combining these two classes can result in a substantial increase in the incidence and severity of side effects, including elevated potassium levels, low blood pressure, kidney damage, cough, and the sometimes fatal allergic reactions. If you have any questions about this, check your medicine cabinet and talk with your doctor.

So the ARBs are safe and effective when used correctly. You know how they work and now you know the things to watch out for.

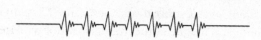

49

Combination Blood Pressure Drugs: Are They Worth It?

There are more than a billion of us walking around on this planet with uncontrolled hypertension. This fact makes the "silent killer" the biggest single contributor to worldwide deaths, and any effort that will help manage this global problem will yield significant benefits. Having effective blood pressure medicines has made a real impact in this area, but more needs to be done. A billion is a big number.

While many of us can achieve our blood pressure goal with a single medicine, most will require two or more drugs to get the job done. In fact, if our BP can initially be controlled with one medicine, the odds are against us that this will always be the case. As time passes, our pressure gradually creeps upward, and the number of us who require more than one medication increases. In fact, several large studies indicate that more than 30 percent of us are on two medications, and more than 20 percent are on three. That's a lot of pills.

Unfortunately, if we have high blood pressure, there's a good chance we have some of the things that to go along with it. Remember the metabolic syndrome—abnormal lipids, elevated glucose, hypertension. All of these conditions frequently require medications, sometimes several. It doesn't take long to need a tote bag to carry all your pill bottles, and you become keenly aware of how difficult it can be to keep everything straight.

Missed doses—lost pills—what do I take when? We welcome anything that can make this process simpler.

Combining multiple blood pressure medicines into a single pill can help accomplish this. It's called a "fixed dose combination" (FDC), with one pill containing two or more medications from different classes. This has proven to be very useful in the management of hypertension, helping to eliminate the possibility of confusion and error. Initially the cost of these combinations was significantly greater than buying the individual components. That's still true for many of them, but as time passes, more become generic and costs drop. That's an important consideration for most of us.

The pharmaceutical companies have made a reasonable effort to provide appropriate combinations of various classes, tailoring them to specific problems and demographics. For example, here are some commonly encountered FDCs:

An ACE inhibitor and a diuretic
Uniretic
Vaseretoc
Lotensin HCT
An ARB and a diuretic
Benicar HCT
Micardis HCT
A beta-blocker and a diuretic
Corzide
And a triple combo—CCB, ARB, and a diuretic
Tribenzor

We'll see that most of the combinations include a diuretic, usually hydrochlorothiazide. There are some limitations with this drug, as we discussed. And there are some limitations with it in combination with any of the other classes.

This combining of blood pressure medicines has exploded over the past few years, with new medications seemingly released each week. The drug companies have managed to tweak the doses in these pills and have come up with multiple combinations. Keep in mind that we have four classes of hypertensive medicines to choose from, with many drugs in each class.

The possible number of mixtures makes our heads spin. Then these new combinations are aggressively promoted as being unique and indispensable. Makes you wonder.

In the next chapter, we'll look at the benefits and drawbacks of these medicines.

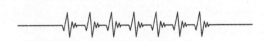

50

The Combination Drugs: The Pros and Cons

We've already mentioned the convenience of taking a single pill instead of two or three. But does this convenience bring with it any other benefits that might offset any increases in cost? The answer here is yes. Let's consider what those might be.

One of the first questions with any new drug or new combination has to do with its effectiveness. Does the medicine work? And does it work as well or better than currently available medicines? Several studies have demonstrated that the effectiveness of fixed-dose combinations is at least equal and sometimes superior to the single medications. So this doesn't seem to be a concern for use of the combinations.

With convenience might come an increased adherence in taking our medications as prescribed. After all, if your blood pressure medicine remains in the bathroom cabinet, it's not going to do you much good. The evidence indicates that the fixed-dose combinations have consistently been shown to increase adherence to a medication plan—something that's obviously important.

Along with this increased adherence comes a reduction in the potential for missed or doubled doses. The use of pill dispensers and reminders helps as well, organizing a day's medications into a.m. or p.m. doses. This handy system is easier to accomplish with fewer pills.

Another interesting benefit of using these combination drugs is an improved perception of an individual's sense of well-being. This might be a little bit of a stretch, but there is some evidence that taking fewer prescription pills has a positive impact on our mental and emotional health. The more pills we take, the less healthy we feel about ourselves. This can lead to a lack or loss of motivation and even depression. It makes sense and is something to think about.

One last benefit of these combos is the reduction in medication side effects. Remember that most of these adverse drug reactions are dose-related—the more of the drug we take, the greater the potential of having a side effect. With fixed-dose combinations, low doses of many of these drugs are available and have been proven to be effective. This results in fewer side effects when compared to using higher dose single drugs.

So there are some advantages and benefits—the pros—when using the combination blood pressure medications. We've considered the cost of these pills as a potentially significant con, but are there others?

Yes. The first have to do with the very nature of taking these combinations. We have to ask and answer the following questions:

- Can my blood pressure be controlled with just one medicine?
- How will I know if one of the medicines is working and the other is not?
- If I have a side effect with this combo, how will we figure out which of the drugs is causing it?

Your physician should be able to answer these questions. Additionally, they will need to determine that none of the drugs in the combination pill will cause a problem with one or more medical conditions you might have (beta-blockers and asthma, for example).

If we keep these things in mind, the cons with these combinations can usually be overcome. One real disadvantage, though, is the current limitation of these medications in one important regard. When we discussed the water pills—specifically the thiazide diuretics—we noted that hydrochlorothiazide (HCTZ) is the most frequently used drug in this class. It's also the most commonly used diuretic in our combination medicines. But it's not the best thiazide diuretic. That would be chlorthalidone. It lasts longer in our system, is more potent than HCTZ, and has been proven to be more cardio-protective than HCTZ. As of this writing, there are only two chlorthalidone combinations on the market—Tenoretic and a new drug that combines chlorthalidone with an ARB. It takes awhile for the pharmaceutical industry to catch up with solid medical research, and this is one of those areas where this needs to happen.

The bottom line here—the combination drugs can be safe and effective, and if the cost is acceptable, they should be a consideration in our efforts to control hypertension.

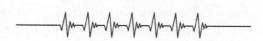

51

The Big Guns:
When All Else Fails

Sometimes we need reinforcements. The battle is drifting in the wrong direction, things aren't working, and we need help—the big guns. First, a couple of definitions are in order. In the ER, we see people whose blood pressures are through the roof—sometimes greater than 200/140 mm Hg. As you can imagine, this gets our attention. This is a *hypertensive emergency*. In fact, if someone's blood pressure is 180/120 or more and they have evidence of the target organ damage we've discussed (cardiac, kidney, or neurologic), they would fall in the same category—a hypertensive emergency. And we're going to get moving and get that pressure down as quickly as we can.

But what if your BP is 180/120 and you don't have any evidence of target organ damage? You might have come to the ER or doctor's office with a sprained ankle or a cut finger. Still an emergency? No, as long as there's no evidence of the problems noted above. This falls into the category of *hypertensive urgency*, and our approach will be much different. This is much more common, and depending upon individual circumstances, we're going to get that pressure down over a period or hours or days. We have a little time here, but some things need to get started.

How does this happen? How does someone's blood pressure get this high, maybe without them even knowing it? There are a couple of circumstances, and in the ER or office, we'll see them all. The first, and maybe most common, is the person who has no clue they have high blood pressure. They're on no medications and are just as surprised as we are when that number passes 180. Then there are those who have hypertension, have medication, but take it only when they feel like it or when they remember. Happens a lot. And finally there are those who have hypertension, may or may not take their medication, but pay no attention to their salt intake. They probably keep a shaker in their pants pocket. But sodium is a serious factor here—an insidious culprit that can rapidly tip the scales and get our blood pressure completely out of whack.

If we're faced with a hypertensive urgency and the individual is already on medication, we'll make the necessary adjustments, try to get their attention, and monitor them closely over the next few days. If they're not on any BP drugs, we'll get some started and monitor them also. Occasionally though, we're faced with someone who regularly takes their medicines, doesn't abuse salt, and who works hard at keeping their blood pressure under control. Yet, they find themselves in this circumstance. Where can we turn for help?

There are a few drugs we can use short-term (longer if absolutely needed) to get things under control. Let's take a look at these.

Clonidine (not to be confused with Klonopin, an antianxiety drug). Clonidine, also known by the brand name Catapres, is an interesting medication. Unlike other hypertensive drugs, the site of its action is in the brain. It does this by stimulating specialized receptors that reduce vascular resistance—relaxing our blood vessels—thus lowering blood pressure. Since the brain is where it exerts its effects, it does some other things here. It's also been found to be useful in the treatment of migraine headaches, anxiety disorders, and even some forms of hyperactivity. Clonidine's calming action is thought to be at least partially responsible for its ability to lower blood pressure. It's potent in doing this, and only a small dose is usually all that's required to help lower a markedly elevated BP. It's given orally, and will take an hour or so to take effect. Some of us may need to use this for extended periods, but the most common circumstance is to discontinue it when our pressure has been stabilized with other medicines.

Hydralazine (Apresoline). This drug has been around for decades and acts by relaxing the smooth muscle in our arteries and smaller arterioles. This action occurs quickly and sometimes can be profound, causing a precipitous drop in our blood pressure. This is dangerous in the elderly and those with heart disease, and can sometimes precipitate angina or even a heart attack. Yet this medication is effective and safe when used carefully. It will get our pressures down quickly, and it has been one of the first-line drugs for the control of hypertension during pregnancy. Other than that important setting, we generally use it sparingly due to its bothersome side effects. These include headaches, heart palpitations, and a rapid heart rate. It's also been known to induce a lupus-like condition with its familiar rash, joint pain, and kidney problems. Rare, but it happens. Hydralazine is a short-term drug to be sure, but it can be lifesaving.

Nitroglycerin and other nitrates. Nitrates have been used for a long time and are well known to most of us. One nitroglycerin tablet under the tongue has saved countless movie heroes through the years, and we still use it today. These drugs cause *venous* dilatation, not arterial as we see with hydralazine and some of our other hypertension medications. By dilating the venous system, it lowers our blood pressure and reduces the work of the heart. That's why it's helpful with angina and with a heart attack. It's also useful in lowering a markedly elevated blood pressure and can be given as a pill, or as that dissolvable tablet under the tongue, or even as a paste applied to the skin. Under the tongue acts the quickest, but its effect in lowering our blood pressure is usually gradual and controlled. These are effective medications and helpful in the setting of hypertensive urgency.

When we considered beta-blockers in an earlier chapter, we also mentioned their sister drugs, the *alpha-blockers*. The alpha-receptor sites, just like the beta sites, are located throughout the body. But they act a little differently, and when blocked, they produce a variety of actions. One of these is the relaxation of some of our blood vessels, leading to a lower blood pressure. They also have been found to be useful in treating panic attacks, anxiety disorders, and even posttraumatic stress disorder (PTSD). And they even help with the treatment of an enlarged prostate. Some examples of these are the following:

Prazosin (Minipress)—especially useful with PTSD
Tamsulosin (Flomax)
Terazosin (Hytrin)—useful with prostate problems

While not necessarily among our big guns, these drugs are effective at lowering blood pressure and useful when our standard medications are not effective. They're another class of hypertensive medicines we can reach for, especially in the setting of some of these other problems.

So there are some of the things we can call on when needed. The main point here is to never need these big guns. We need to take our medicine regularly, pay attention to our salt intake, and stay on top of our blood pressures. But the reinforcements are there.

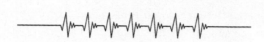

52

Children and Adolescents (Yes, They Get High Blood Pressure Too)

Most of us either have or one day will have children. Maybe even grand-children. And if not, there are probably significant youngsters in our lives. We usually don't think of these young people as having the diseases that affect those of us more advanced in years—but they do. Kidney disease, diabetes, and hypertension.

High blood pressure frequently begins in childhood and adolescence, and can lead to the early onset of cardiovascular disease. Some of these changes include the development of atherosclerosis ("hardening of the arteries") and evidence of thickening and enlargement of the heart itself.

How does this happen? How does a ten-year-old develop high blood pressure? As with adults, we divide hypertension into two types: primary (we used to call this *essential*) and secondary. We don't know what causes primary hypertension, but the secondary type has a diagnosable and usu-ally treatable cause. This could be kidney problems such as stones, small kidneys, congenital defects, or the result of trauma. Thyroid and adrenal diseases, as well as diabetes, can also cause secondary hypertension. The list of causes is extensive and includes medications, blood vessel abnor-malities, and certain cancers.

The difference between children and adults is that secondary hyper-tension is much more common in young people (more than 75 percent) while primary hypertension is the cause in more than 90 percent of hypertensive adults. This consideration is important, since we want to identify those children who have a cause for their high blood pressure, find it, and eliminate it.

Since finding the cause of secondary hypertension is so important, what are some tipoffs, some factors that might point us in that direction? Here's what we know. Secondary hypertension should be considered if a child has one or more of the following:

- the onset of high blood pressure before puberty, usually before the age of ten years

- a sudden elevation in blood pressure from levels that were previously normal

- a slender child who doesn't have a family history of high blood pressure

- a significantly elevated BP (this would be stage 2, discussed below)

- a past history of kidney infections

- a family history of chronic kidney disease or congenital renal problems

- findings of elevated blood pressure in the arms but not the legs (this is suggestive of a narrowing of the aorta and is potentially correctable)

Now let's take a look at how we define high blood pressure in those under the age of twenty. It's a little different than in adults. We considered earlier that some experts view systolic hypertension to be more significant in adults than an elevated diastolic number. With children and adolescents, both of these pressures are of equal importance. Another difference is that normal BP levels in this group are based on percentiles. If you've taken a child to the pediatrician's office, you've probably watched the nurse plot measurements of height and weight on a standardized graph. The same is true for blood pressure, and it's based on age and height.

As a couple of examples, consider an eight-year-old boy who's at the fiftieth percentile in height. His levels would be as follows:

Normal BP—less than 112/73
Prehypertension—up to 116/78
Stage 1 hypertension—up to 121/83
Stage 2 hypertension—greater than 128/91

The first thing you probably noticed is how low these numbers appear. For an adult 121/83 would be a great pressure. Not so in this eight-year-old boy.

And how about a fourteen-year-old girl, also at the fiftieth percentile in height? Here are her numbers:

Normal BP—less than 122/78
Prehypertension—up to 126/82
Stage 1 hypertension—up to 131/87
Stage 2 hypertension—greater than 138/95

Again, these are not crazy-high numbers. Yet stage 2 hypertension carries with it a lot of long-term consequences.

These categories are important for how concerned we are with a particular BP reading and how we treat this problem. Other factors that enter into our management have to do with what's called "comorbidities"—evidence of target organ damage, just like in adults. These would be heart problems (that thickened heart muscle noted above), neurological changes, and evidence of kidney damage. If any of these are present, a bunch of red flags should go up and the approach to treatment becomes more aggressive.

If a young person falls into the prehypertensive category, our initial strategy should be nondrug intervention. Lifestyle changes. These are pretty much the same as those described for adults. Regular exercise is encouraged, as is a reduction in weight to a normal level. We need to know if the child is smoking and make every effort to be sure this stops. Salt restriction is critical, just as it is with adults.

Here's something interesting I recently came across. A study was done of newborns, dividing them into two groups—one group received a diet containing normal amounts of sodium and the other was placed on a low-salt diet. These infants were followed for six months, at which time the low-salt group was found to have significantly lower blood pressures. Fifteen years later, this difference persisted, regardless of the type of diet beyond the six months of the study. That's impressive, and while too late for you and me, it's not too late to consider for a lot of newborns and yet-to-be-borns.

If blood pressure levels don't normalize in those with prehypertension, some experts would consider starting low-dose medications. Certainly those with stage 1 and 2 hypertension will probably need medication, along with lifestyle modifications. And any child having evidence of target organ damage should have their pressures lowered into the normal range as quickly as possible. There are some differences regarding medication choices when it comes to treating hypertension in children and adolescents, and most physicians would advise involving a pediatrician skilled in this area. It's important, and if undetected or untreated, the damage caused in childhood can last a lifetime—and shorten it.

So if you have children or grandchildren, you or somebody's gotta know their numbers.

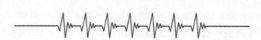

53

Special Circumstances

I'm thankful that for many of us, the approach to the control of high blood pressure and the choice of medication is straightforward. That's the case with Dave Jernigan. He doesn't have any unusual or complicating conditions that might make his management more difficult. He does have elevated lipids and is on medication for that, but that's something we can work around.

But not everyone is Dave Jernigan, and there are things that can prove challenging for a lot of us. These special medical conditions require careful consideration of the appropriate medicines to use and specific things to watch for, and they may even cause us to change our blood pressure goals. Let's take a look at these. They're very common, and you might find yourself included in one or more of these groups.

Special Medical Conditions

Diabetes. Individuals with diabetes will usually require two or more drugs to reach their target blood pressure goal of less than 140/90. All of the major groups are effective in reducing the risk of cardiovascular disease and stroke, while the ACE inhibitors and ARBs are helpful for kidney function. They slow the progression of diabetic kidney disease and reduce the loss of protein in the urine.

Ischemic Heart Disease (Angina). This is the most common form of target organ damage in people with high blood pressure. Under some circumstances, the beta-blockers can be helpful here, as well as the calcium channel blockers. If an individual has had a heart attack, ACE inhibitors should be considered, along with aggressive lipid management and daily aspirin.

Heart Failure. This occurs when the muscles of the heart are not functioning properly and the heart is unable to keep up with the oxygen needs of the body. Management of high blood pressure in the face of heart failure can be tricky, and your physician needs to have experience in this area. ACE inhibitors are frequently used, along with spironolactone, a different acting medication that blocks a hormone produced by the adrenal gland.

Chronic Kidney Disease. This is another of the target organ damage problems that we frequently encounter. The kidneys lose their ability to properly filter the blood and an important waste product—creatinine—begins to accumulate. Hypertension is a frequent cause of kidney disease and is almost always found in those suffering with it. Treatment includes aggressive blood pressure management with ACE inhibitors and ARBs, though these drugs can themselves cause a small rise in creatinine levels. We just have to watch this closely and be aware of potential pitfalls. Should kidney function continue to decline, the loop diuretics (Lasix) are usually required to maintain adequate urine production.

The Metabolic Syndrome. Remember the components here: obesity, elevated triglycerides, a low HDL, glucose intolerance, and high blood pressure. We're not sure which is the cart and which is the horse, but the management of hypertension in this syndrome is one of the cornerstones of treatment. This is a cascade of bad things and requires aggressive targeting of several aspects of our health, focusing on lifestyle changes. All four of the first-line classes of blood pressure drugs can be used here.

Hypertension in Older Persons. High blood pressure is found in more than two-thirds of us over the age of sixty-five. It turns out that this population also has the lowest rates of blood pressure control, so this is a significant concern. Treatment in these individuals is tailored in a similar fashion to those younger, though initial doses may need to be lowered in order to prevent problems. Ultimately, most will require standard doses and multiple drugs to meet their BP goal.

Dementia. This is a growing challenge, and we know that dementia (such as Alzheimer's) and other forms of cognitive impairment occur more commonly in people with high blood pressure. Some studies indicate that effective control of hypertension can reduce the progression of these life-robbing diseases. No one class of drugs appears to be better than another in this instance, and a standard approach is usually in order.

Hypertension in Women. This represents a little more than half of us— my wife would say the better and more important half. There are some significant considerations to keep in mind with women being treated for high blood pressure. Oral contraceptives may cause an increase in blood pressure, and this risk increases the longer the contraceptive is taken. Women who become pregnant or who are planning on doing so must avoid ACE inhibitors and ARBs, as they have the potential to cause fetal defects. Methyldopa, one of the older drugs, and the beta-blockers would be the choices here.

Minorities. We have a problem in this country with the control of hypertension in various minority populations. For instance, the lowest incidence of treatment and control is found in Mexican-Americans and Native Americans. And we know that the incidence, severity, and impact of high blood pressure is increased in African-Americans. For some unknown reason, these individuals don't respond as well to single therapy with beta-blockers, ACE inhibitors, and ARBs, yet they do with the diuretics and calcium channel blockers. Most will respond to combination therapy, which needs to include adequate doses of a diuretic.

Hypertension in Children and Adolescents. As we considered in the previous chapter, high blood pressure does occur in our young people, and it needs to be identified and treated. Lifestyle changes (weight management, diet, and especially exercise) are central to this effort, but blood pressure medications may be needed and are generally the same as those used in adults. We frequently get questions about athletic participation for young people who have high blood pressure. If the problem has been evaluated (from a cardiac, kidney, and endocrine perspective), physical activity should be encouraged, particularly since long-term and vigorous exercise can help lower blood pressure.

Additional Factors to Keep in Mind

- Thiazide diuretics can be helpful in slowing the progression of osteoporosis.
- Calcium channel blockers might be useful in the treatment

of Raynaud's syndrome—a blanching of the fingers with cold exposure.

- Beta-blockers are beneficial in the treatment of certain cardiac rhythm disturbances (atrial fibrillation), specific types of tremors, and migraine headaches, but as previously noted, have fallen out of favor as first-line blood pressure medicines.

- Thiazide diuretics can worsen or precipitate gout and can cause low sodium and potassium levels.

- Beta-blockers should be avoided in persons with asthma or other types of reactive airway disease, since they can cause an acute attack.

- ACE inhibitors are a known cause of chronic cough and can be associated with swelling (edema) of the face and tongue. Once this happens, these drugs should never be used again. For some reason, this type of edema occurs three to four times more frequently in African-Americans.

Resistant Hypertension

One last but important special consideration in the treatment of high blood pressure is something called *resistant hypertension,* and it's just what you'd think it would be—blood pressure that can't be controlled. In the technical sense, it's "failure to reach BP goal in patients who are adhering to full doses of an appropriate three-drug regimen that includes a diuretic." The first and most important step is to identify known but possibly subtle causes of high blood pressure. These include the following:

- undiagnosed kidney disease

- sleep apnea

- chronic steroid (prednisone) therapy

- tumors that produce epinephrine-like chemicals (rare)

- thyroid disease

- diseases of the adrenal gland

- renal artery diseases (narrowing of the blood vessels)

After these have been ruled out, the challenge remains to unearth a potential cause for this lack of response to treatment. Here are some of the things that need to be explored:

- excess sodium intake (a frequent offender)
- inadequate diuretic therapy
- inadequate doses of medications
- nonadherence to treatment (sometimes difficult to determine)
- oral contraceptives
- anabolic steroids (again, sometimes difficult to elicit)
- over-the-counter supplements (ma huang, ephedra)
- excess alcohol intake
- cocaine, amphetamines, other illicit drugs
- inappropriate drug combinations (physician-induced)
- NSAIDs—ibuprofen, naproxen
- over-the-counter decongestants
- over-the-counter appetite suppressants (many have been found to contain varying amounts of amphetamine-type drugs)
- licorice (This exerts a hormonal effect on your kidneys, causing an elevation in blood pressure. It takes a good bit of it, but it's something to keep in mind.)

As you can see, managing high blood pressure is not as simple as "Here, take this pill and we'll see you in a couple of months." There's a lot to think about, and it can be challenging. But if you and your physician are motivated and you work at it, you can get there.

54

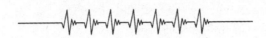

You Gotta Know Your Numbers

A Ticking Time Bomb

"Congratulations, Chad. Looks like you've finally done it."

The fifty-one-year-old slouched on the exam table and cocked his head at me as I walked into the exam room.

"What's that, Doc?"

I had known Chad Hennigar since we moved to Rock Hill twenty years earlier. He was an investment banker and we occasionally played golf together.

"You've finally achieved every major risk factor for developing heart disease."

He chuckled and shook his head. "Well isn't that somethin'. I know I'm overweight and my cholesterol is high. And last visit you told me about my blood sugar."

"Diabetes," I said. "Your diabetes."

"Alright, but I've been taking the medicine you prescribed and tried to cut down on my carbs. No more ice cream before I go to bed—at least not every night."

It was my turn to shake my head. Chad was incorrigible and quite a challenge. But we were going to continue working on this.

"You said *all* the risk factors, Doc. I've cut down on my smoking, so what else is there?"

"Well, you're a male—that one was easy—and you're over fifty."

"Just barely," he said. "Only fifty-one."

"Okay, just barely. But that's another factor. And now—" I opened his chart and pointed to today's vital signs. "Now your blood pressure is elevated to the point where we need to do something about it."

He sighed. "How high is elevated?"

"It's been slowly edging upward for several months. We've talked about that, Chad, and about cutting out your salt and losing some weight. That hasn't happened, and now your pressure is 150 over 98. Not a dangerous level, but we're going to have to deal with it."

Another long sigh. "Does this mean medication?"

"We've tried working on your lifestyle, but that's just not happening. This is one of the most important risk factors for you—maybe the most important—and we can do something about it. So yes, it's going to mean starting some medication."

"I'm already taking that statin drug you gave me, and the fish oil and niacin. Another pill—really? What if we try a couple more months with a diet and cutting down on the salt and exercising? What if—"

"Chad, do you really think that's going to work?"

He stared at the floor and didn't say anything. Finally he shook his head and looked up at me. "No, you're right. Just give me a prescription and I'll start taking it."

We talked for a while about what I thought would be the best type of medicine for him to start, when to take it, and any potential side effects to watch out for. And we talked again about the lifestyle changes he needed to make.

"And get rid of the cigarettes," I told him as I opened the exam room door. "Don't just cut down some. You've got to totally quit, once and for all."

"I hear you. When do I come back?"

"Let's make it in three or four weeks, and see how the medicine's working," I answered.

"Fine. I'll see you then."

Chad's wife, Cheryl, was with him at his next appointment. She was standing by his side when I walked into the room.

"Hey, Robert," she said. "What good news do you have for us today?"

I sat in front of them and opened his chart. I didn't see any good news. "Well, it looks like you've gained three pounds in the last month, Chad. And your blood pressure isn't any better. Maybe a couple of points worse."

Cheryl shot a glance at her husband. "That shouldn't come as a surprise, should it, Chad? Have you been taking your blood pressure medicine or did you stop again?"

"Again?" I asked, looking at my flushing friend.

"We had the prescription filled the day you gave it to him," Cheryl explained. "And started it the next morning. He tried it for a week or so but didn't like the way it made him feel. And he stopped taking it."

"How did it make you feel, Chad? What problems were you having?"

"It wasn't exactly *problems*," he muttered. "It's just that…"

"It's just that his friends told him it would interfere with his love life," Cheryl said. "I told him our love life wouldn't matter much if he died from a stroke or a heart attack."

"She's got a point there, Chad." I smiled and tapped his chart with my pen. "So you really weren't having any problems with the medicine?"

"No, I guess not," he answered. "I guess it's just the idea of taking another pill. I feel like an old man."

"That's the whole point, Chad. We want you to get to the point of *being* an old man."

We talked again about his risk factors, and I stressed that he was a walking time bomb and needed to change some things. Chad promised he would do better, and Cheryl promised to help.

I'm not sure if Chad ever started his blood pressure medicine again. When Cheryl and I talked a month later at the funeral, she wasn't sure either.

"He told me he was taking it, but I wasn't going to snoop and count his pills. I almost did, that last morning when he headed out to the golf course."

One of his friends told me what had happened. Chad had shanked an approach shot into the greenside bunker on number nine. He climbed into the trap, scattered sand everywhere with his shot, then clutched his chest and collapsed.

Boom.

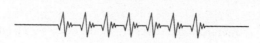

55

Don't Be Misled

More doctors smoke Camels than any other cigarette.

Some of us may be old enough to remember a few of these advertisements. The tobacco companies recruited babies and even Santa Claus to ply their wares. In one ad, Jolly Ole Saint Nick admonishes us to "guard against throat-scratch" by smoking Pall Malls.

It's a good thing we've gotten so much smarter now. None of us would ever fall for that kind of...Well, not so fast. There have been hucksters aplenty for a lot of years, and we have shelled out a lot of hard-earned dollars for their highly touted products. Here are a couple of examples, some of which may surprise you.

The makers of Listerine, named after the famous and nonhuckster scientist Joseph Lister, claimed early on that its mouthwash cured a wide range of medical conditions, including sore throats, the common cold, coughs, and even dandruff. It took several decades for the Federal Trade Commission (FTC) to order the company to stop making such claims, having proved that the product was no more effective in the treatment of colds than gargling with warm salt water.

And then there was Dr. Koch's Cure-All—a surefire remedy for allergies, infections of various kinds, tuberculosis, and even cancer. It wasn't until 1948 that the FDA tested this "remedy" and determined that it contained nothing more than distilled water. Yet countless individuals had spent countless dollars and precious time on this worthless cure-all.

The promotion of these dubious wares didn't end in the middle of the last century. Only a few years ago, several patients would come to our office complaining of facial pain, drainage, and fever—symptoms of a possible sinus infection.

"I don't understand it, Doc. I tried that new Airborne stuff and I still got sick."

You might remember these over-the-counter chewable tablets or gummies, or (don't raise your hand) might have even tried them. "Designed by a school teacher," it was purported to prevent colds and even boost your immune system. A couple of lawsuits later, we know that this product was falsely advertised, possessing none of the asserted benefits. Yet millions of dollars and a lot of time was spent by people looking for some help and hoping they had found some. Unfortunately, this stuff is still available though still unproven.

Lastly (and again, don't raise your hand), how many of us have tried the weight-loss product Sensa? What could be easier than sprinkling these crystals on top of your food and watching the weight disappear? No dieting, no exercise, just this magical dust that suppresses appetite and melts away those pounds—an average of thirty in six months. Too good to be true? Of course, and the FTC knows it. The makers have been charged with deceptive advertising, but it's still on the market and still with absolutely no evidence that supports its wondrous claims.

Curious about any of these products? Just check them out on the Internet.

Ah, the Internet. P.T. Barnum must be turning over in his grave, trying to return and get a shot at the vast and pervasive peddling potential of being online. What a great opportunity! You can offer things for sale that have absolutely no value or make any claims you want with complete disregard for their veracity.

But how are we to know? How are we to separate the wheat from the chaff, especially when it comes to matters concerning our health and physical well-being? That's a significant problem, and it's becoming more difficult. You can find any possible opinion online, presented as fact, maybe even as gospel. So what are we to do? How can we be effectively armed to avoid the next Dr. Koch's Cure-All? There's hope here, and some advice.

First, when you're trying to find information about a medication or diagnosis or anything medical, pay attention to the bottom line. If it involves buying something, it's time to exit that website.

Second, check out the source of the information. Is this something or someone reputable? Sounds easy enough, but several of my patients will quote famous TV doctors, and the information they have been given is frequently just flat wrong. Again, check the bottom line.

And last, if some issue is important to you, check out a couple of good resources before coming to a conclusion or making a decision. But where are we going to find those resources and who can be trusted? Here are some of the places I look.

For basic information that is quick, factual, and straightforward:

Mayo Clinic (www.mayoclinic.org)
WebMD (www.webmd.com)

For a more in-depth look at specific subjects:

American Academy of Family Physicians (www.aafp.org)
National Institutes of Health (nih.gov)
National Center for Biotechnology Information (NCBI)
(www.ncbi.nlm.nih.gov)
PubMed (pubmed.gov)
Centers for Disease Control and Prevention (www.cdc.gov)

For accurate and interesting information, and a source that's searched by many physicians:

Wikipedia (en.wikipedia.org)

A great resource that stays current with the most recent research and information—mainly intended for physicians and other healthcare providers:

UpToDate (www.uptodate.com)
(Some basic content is available for free, but full access requires purchasing a subscription.)

So there are some places to turn if you have a question about a health issue. And if you're still confused or not yet satisfied, contact me at robert lesslie.com. I may not always have the answer, but I'll always have an opinion.

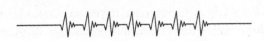

It's All About Balance

I included this in my book 60 Ways to Lower Your Cholesterol. *Since that book's release, several readers and friends have made meaningful suggestions and comments about this chapter, encouraging me to include them here. I have gratefully done so.*

The sweet spot. We're all searching for it—some without realizing.

If you play golf, you know it instantly. You make contact with the ball and it's...perfect. All you've ever tried to do with a golf club has come together in this one moment, this one swing. You don't need to look up—you know where that round white object is headed.

The same is true for a tennis player. Racket meets ball and you just know. All of your power and accuracy come together in that one rare instant. Perfect.

And there's the four-part a cappella singing group. The musical piece flows to a critical moment and there it is—a chord whose harmony stirs your very soul, resonates within your entire being, transports you out of this everyday world. It doesn't matter whether you're one of the singers or someone in the audience. It's perfect.

And then reality. We stand over that golf ball, swing as hard as we can, and watch a duck hook fly out of bounds. We swing our tennis racket too early and at the wrong angle, and that fuzzy ball sails over the fence. And the baritone, approaching that climactic harmony, is suddenly moved to pursue his own unwritten musical line, and our teeth are instantly set on edge.

The sweet spot. Forever sought after. Forever elusive.

We seek that same elusive sweet spot in our lives as well. We live in an age of distraction, constantly bombarded by an ever-expanding array of diversions. Those distractions make it very difficult if not impossible for us to focus on the things and people and moments that are important. It's an internal struggle as well. Our attention is fractured by ever-shifting hopes and dreams, plans and schemes, inward hurts and wild imaginings.

We're a jumbled mess, aren't we?

Should we ever find this *balance*, what would it look like? As are many of us, I'm a visual learner—you know, "one picture is worth a thousand words." I've attached some diagrams in an attempt to convey how this might appear in our lives. It's never this simple, but we need to start somewhere.

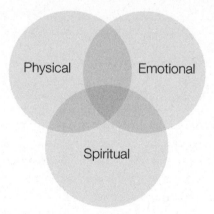

You'll note the three areas here. Let's talk about these.

The *physical* part of our lives is just that. This is largely what we deal with in our medical clinic every day—injuries, illnesses, or the desire for better health and disease prevention. We focus on what we can see and feel, and that's not a bad thing. We *need* to stay as healthy as we can for as long as we can, and to heal as quickly as possible when injured or sick. And we need to pay attention to things that can adversely affect our health, such as an elevated blood pressure.

All of this is important and it's okay. It's when this area of our lives becomes unbalanced that things go wrong. We focus too much on our bodies or on how we look, or we become preoccupied with some vague symptoms that must be the first signs of a terminal illness. That circle grows larger and overwhelms the other two. In this illustration, you can see how we can easily become detached from our spiritual being, completely obsessed with our bodies and health.

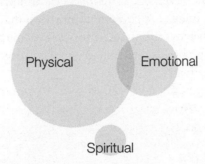

We've even learned to dissociate ourselves from potentially painful emotions and from the "still small voice" that patiently whispers in our ear. We are dogged in our pursuit of physical comfort and pleasure. Nothing new here—we've been chasing these rainbows for thousands of years.

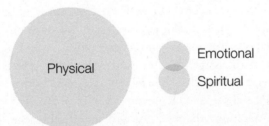

Some of us have even developed the ability to compartmentalize these three areas of our lives, encouraged by a culture that is becoming more and more detached, hedonistic, and focused on the individual.

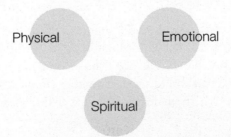

This brings us to our *emotional* part. We are certainly passionate and sensitive creatures. I've lived with two teenage daughters, and the emotional roller coaster was like Disney's Space Mountain but at twice the speed—up, down, sideways, and most of it in the dark. Anyway, some experts liken this to a colorful, interconnected cluster of feelings: love, pity, outrage, affection, happiness, suffering, self-confidence, shyness, anger, guilt, depression, pride, despair, regret, surprise, wonder, and many more. No wonder we're all over the place. It's easy to imagine how our emotional lives can quickly become distorted and out of balance.

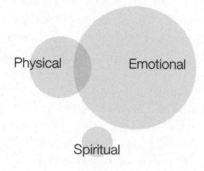

We are all too easily overwhelmed by grief and anger, blinded by love, or diminished by shyness and disappointment. We know our emotional life impacts our physical being—weight gain or loss, lack of energy, obsession with real and imagined diseases. And we know the effects too much stress can have on our health. We've looked at the effect it can have on our blood pressure, and we know it's a very real contributor to heart attacks and strokes, in addition to being the cause of inexplicable aches, pains, and multiple complaints. We've even come to understand that this chronic stress can raise our lipid levels and promote the formation of dangerous plaques in our arteries.

When our emotional lives are not in balance, bad things happen. We see it every day.

That leaves us with the *spiritual* component of our lives. What are we talking about here? This is that deepest place in our innermost beings, separate yet connected to our physical and emotional selves. It's not just a feel-good spot—that would make it another emotion. It's something altogether different. It's been described as that void created within us that longs to be filled by our Creator. Most of us would call this our *soul.* C.S. Lewis describes it this way: "You don't have a soul. You *are* a soul. You have a body."

We neglect this part of our lives at our own peril, becoming preoccupied with our physical bodies or driven by every changing emotional wind.

Much of the time we are that jumbled mess I spoke of earlier, and our lives look like what we see when we look through a kaleidoscope, only nowhere near as pretty. But behind those beautiful colors and shapes are hard, sharp, ever-shifting shards of glass—just as it is within each of us. It's a tough place to be, and we seek ways to find balance and to find peace.

Finding that balance—that sweet spot—is a lifelong journey. But it's not an impossible one. Notice the chair in the center of the diagram below. Actually it's a throne, and it's the *key* to our balance and peace.

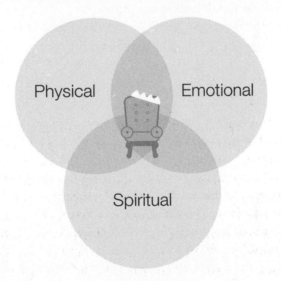

This is the very center of our lives, the very seat of our being. And it poses a question that is critical for each of us. And each of us, whether we acknowledge it or not, answers this question every day of our lives. *Who sits on that throne?* If we put ourselves there, we're bound for failure. If we're the captain of our ship, the master of our destiny, well...good luck. And if we place another person there, we're headed for disaster as well. We all suffer from the limitations of being human, and we will hurt and disappoint each other—even our friends and loved ones.

Here's where we're constantly playing musical chairs, circling that throne each day, waiting for the music to stop and see who jumps into that seat—who's going to be in charge of our lives. It's usually us, or because of some circumstance or crisis, it could be a friend or loved one. But that will only be temporary. Our desire, our nature is to be in that chair.

But someone else could occupy that throne—the Man from Galilee. He stands patiently waiting for each of us, waiting for us to choose. He knows our hearts, and understands what pastor and author A.W. Tozer said: "Every man lives by faith, the nonbeliever as well as the saint; the one by faith in natural laws and the other by faith in God."

I chose faith in God, the author of our natural laws. With the balance, centeredness, and peace that He brings from His presence on that throne, we're able to handle whatever this brief life throws our way—whether it be physical challenges or emotional turmoil.

Balance. The sweet spot. It's where we were created to live.

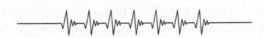

Frequently Asked Questions

By now, you've probably got some questions—maybe things you've been wondering about for a while. Here are some of the more frequent (and interesting) queries from our patients.

Q: Once I start blood pressure medicine, will I have to take it for the rest of my life?

The answer here is a straightforward yes and maybe. Once started on blood pressure medication, most people will need to continue it for the rest of their lives. Keep in mind that the normal aging process brings with it many unwanted changes, including a gradual increase in our blood pressures. And we all know how hard it is to give up bad and unhealthy habits. However, if sufficiently motivated to improve our lifestyles—more exercise, no smoking, achieving and maintaining our ideal weight, really restricting our salt intake—it might be possible to stop our BP medicine. This will need to be carefully coordinated with your physician, but yes, it's possible. Maybe.

Q: What's the best time of day to take my medication, morning or night?

I'm glad you asked this question. A lot of people wonder about this, and it turns out to be important. For a long time, we didn't think it made any difference when you took these medicines. The only consistent advice was not to take your fluid pill right before going to bed. Not unless you wanted to get up several times during the night and risk falling over the dog.

We now know that aside from those fluid pills (still good advice to take these in the morning), your other blood pressure medicines should be taken at night, before you go to bed. From a statistical standpoint, more heart attacks and strokes occur in the early morning hours—frequently upon arising—and are thought to be due at least in part to a sudden rise in uncontrolled blood pressure. If your medicine was taken the morning before, it has most likely left your system and left you unprotected. Some of the long-acting drugs have helped here, yet this continues to be our most vulnerable time of day. Take your pills before bed or, as an option, take half your daily dosage in the morning and half at night.

Q: The guy at the health-food store recommended some stuff for my blood pressure. What do you think?

It all depends on the stuff. There are a few things that might help, but most of the claims by the manufacturers of these supplements are unfounded. They haven't gone to the trouble and expense to do the necessary research to prove their effectiveness. Or the research might have been done and demonstrated no benefit—maybe even some harm. Yet they continue to be on the shelves of your health-food store because no one's really watching. There's very little oversight in this important and costly area of our healthcare.

You can find out what you need to know by going to: www.nccam.nih .gov/health/herbsataglance.htm.

Q: My aunt told me to drink a tablespoon of vinegar every night and my blood pressure would be fine. Is she crazy?

You'll have to answer the last part, but I can tell you about vinegar. There have been many claims regarding the health benefits of regularly consuming apple (white) vinegar. Lowering cholesterol, losing weight, controlling diabetes, and lowering blood pressure. To date, there is no good evidence that supports any of these claims. On the other hand, white vinegar is effective in removing clogs from drains, breaking down glue for easy removal, and helping strip wallpaper. Should you decide to give it a try for medicinal purposes, be aware that it can attack the enamel of your teeth, causing cavities and sensitivity.

Q: I read where kosher salt is better for you than the regular kind. What do you think?

This is the orthopedic conundrum, only repackaged.

"Mrs. Jones, the X-ray shows little Billy's wrist is fractured."

"Thank heavens! At least it's not broken or cracked."

It's all the same. Kosher salt, sea salt, black salt, Himalayan pink salt, Celtic salt, regular table salt—they're all pretty much equivalent when it comes to their sodium content. There might be some slight variations in contaminants and trace amounts of minerals such as calcium, magnesium, and potassium, but when it comes to your blood pressure and health, there's not a grain of difference.

Q: I read that ibuprofen is bad for your blood pressure, but naproxen is okay. What do you think?

I think, once again, don't believe everything you read. You're right about the ibuprofen. It's one of our nonsteroidal anti-inflammatory drugs (NSAIDs) and it can raise our blood pressure as well as worsen some other cardiovascular risks. But the same is true for *all* the NSAIDs, including naproxen. If you have high blood pressure, you'll need to avoid these drugs. A baby aspirin (81mg) is also an NSAID, but there's no evidence connecting it with worsening hypertension. And for the record, acetaminophen is not an NSAID, nor does it interfere with the control of our BP.

Q: One of my friends said I'll have to give up coffee now that I'm on blood pressure medicine. Is that true?

This is tough for me, because I'm an avid coffee drinker, regularly consuming anywhere from two to six cups per day. The most current evidence indicates that caffeine can cause an acute rise in blood pressure, but not to excessive levels, and then it normalizes over the next half hour or so. This response is seen less frequently in those of us who are accustomed to drinking coffee or tea. If you regularly drink coffee and your blood pressure is normal, you should be fine.

It might be reasonable to conduct a home trial. Check your blood pressure, drink a cup of your favorite brew, and then repeat your pressure in fifteen or twenty minutes. If your systolic pressure goes up by more than

10 points, you may be caffeine sensitive. If the rise is less than this, you're probably okay. It would be a good idea to discuss these findings with your physician.

Q: If I get my pressure under control, can I stop taking medicine? And if so, can I stop cold turkey?

Not just yet, and no. As we considered in our first question, it may be possible to stop taking blood pressure medicine if you have achieved your goal and adjusted your lifestyle. You'll want to be sure you maintain your weight (assuming this has happened) and can continue your other lifestyle changes. Then work with your physician, making sure she advises you along the way. As to *how* to stop, most medications will need to be tapered—usually over two or three weeks—while your pressure is being carefully monitored. This is especially true for the beta-blockers, since stopping cold turkey with some of these can precipitate serious problems, including a heart attack or worse.

Q: My nephew is in premed, and he told me as long as one of my blood pressure numbers was okay, I'd be fine. Do you agree with that?

Say what? Where does your nephew go to school? Of course this is not okay. While it's true there is something called "systolic hypertension"— a condition where our systolic pressure is elevated while our diastolic remains in or near the normal range—this usually occurs as we grow older, it's still serious, and it's something most experts would address. Otherwise, we're going to target *both* of our numbers, keeping in mind that elevations in our systolic and diastolic pressures each bring their own set of problems and complications.

Q: I'm about to have a life-insurance physical and don't want to tell them I take blood pressure medicine. Is there any way they can find out?

Remember what Mark Twain once said: "If you tell the truth, you don't have to remember anything." That's still good advice, aside from the fact that we should always strive to be honest. In this case, you'd better be. Tests can be done (usually on a urine specimen) to determine the presence of several classes of blood pressure medicines, as well as some of the statins. You'll find yourself better off by accurately noting your current medications than should you be caught in an intentional deception. Don't find yourself trapped in that tangled web.

Q: *The nurse at my doctor's office says there's no difference between using a regular size BP cuff or a large one. As you can see, I've got big arms. Does it really matter what size the cuff is?*

Of course it does. If the cuff is too small, your pressure is going to be over-estimated. And if too large, the reading will be lower than the actual numbers. Remember, the cuff needs to be placed with its lower edge one inch above the elbow, and it should cover two-thirds of the upper arm. Make sure this is done correctly.

Q: *Everyone in my family has high blood pressure—going back as many generations as I know about. I'm going to have it, so that's that, and there's nothing I can do.*

Is there a question here or just a statement of futility? It's true that genetics play a significant role in most areas of our lives (nature versus nurture), and our blood pressures are no exception. We are beginning to learn more about this important area, and we do see a trend of hypertension within families and close relatives. While its familial presence should alert you to the possibility of developing high blood pressure, there's no cause for despair. Rather, this should be viewed as a challenge, something to be managed and overcome. So yes, you *can* do something about it.

Q: *Doc, I read your book about lowering cholesterol. You talk about your faith, and I was wondering how you balance that with being a physician? How do you combine your faith with your science?*

I'm glad you asked that question, because it's the easiest one yet. Francis Bacon (1561–1626) might have said it best.

"Little knowledge of science makes a man an atheist,
but in-depth study of science makes him a believer in God."

The psalmist was right—we *are* fearfully and wonderfully made (Psalm 139).

58

Victory!

Dave was beaming. "Did you see my numbers, Doc? Pretty good, aren't they?" He pointed to the clipboard in my hand, then handed me a small notebook, opened to a page with a long list of numbers and times. "And take a look at that."

I had already seen the BP on his chart—118/78. I was impressed. In his notebook were columns of recorded blood pressures, each with the time of day noted beside it. He had marked with an asterisk any pressure over 130/90. I scanned three pages—more than seventy-five readings—and saw only three asterisks.

"Great work, Dave." I closed the notebook and gave it back to him. "Tell me how you did it. What's worked best for you?"

"He's been working out like a triathlete." Lisa stood in the corner of the room, smiling at her husband. "And he won't touch a speck of salt. He's always looking over my shoulder in the kitchen, making sure I don't sneak some into his food."

"I'm not that bad. But I am paying attention to the salt, just like you advised. And I'm exercising more, but I'm no fanatic."

"Whatever you're doing, Dave, it's working." I closed his record and dropped it to the countertop beside me. "And how about your medication? Any problems with it or any side effects?"

"Nope, none at all. No fatigue or anything. I feel great."

"And there's no problem with our love life," Lisa added from across the room.

Dave blushed and grinned. "No problems there, either."

"Alrighty then," I said, standing. "It looks like we're where we need to be. Just keep doing what you're doing, and we'll see you again in six months."

"There *is* one more thing, Doc. We've been at this for seven or eight months, and I've lost a few pounds with all this exercise and the new diet, low carbs and all. But I want to lose another ten or so and I just can't seem to get them off. Have you got any ideas? What can I do?"

I sat down again, crossed my legs, and leaned back. It would take some work, but I had some ideas. Together we would find a way to lose those ten pounds.

"Let's talk about that, Dave."

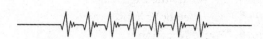

59

Putting It All Together

If you're one of the millions of us with a higher-than-healthy blood pressure, or if you want to give yourself the best chance of avoiding this problem, now's the time to do something about it. Now's the time to get started. It might seem a daunting task, but it can be done.

We've covered a lot of important material in these pages—things I hope you'll refer to as you travel this path of lowering your blood pressure. In an effort to make sense out of all this information, I've organized the key chapters that deal with specific topics.

1. First, you've *got* to know your numbers. High blood pressure *is* the silent killer, but it doesn't have to be. Have your pressure checked at your doctor's office or with a home monitor—before it's too late.

   Chapter 2, "Just Barely"
   Chapter 14, "It's Getting a Little Frosty"
   Chapter 28, "The Sentinel"
   Chapter 37, "Heart Don't Fail Me Now"
   Chapter 54, "A Ticking Time Bomb"

2. Understand what these numbers mean.

   Chapter 7, "Plumbing 101: Basic Blood Pressure Physiology"
   Chapter 8, "The Numbers: What Do They Mean?"

3. Be convinced this is important—even critical to your health and well-being. It's all about knowledge and motivation, then putting those two together.

Chapter 4, "So What's the Big Deal?"
Chapter 5, "The Metabolic Syndrome"
Chapter 6, "You're Not Alone"

4. Take a hard look at your lifestyle and make the changes necessary to improve your blood pressure and overall health.

Chapter 15, "Getting Started"
Chapter 16, "Don't DASH Off: Your Diet as a Weapon Against High Blood Pressure"
Chapter 17, "The Low-Carb Approach"
Chapter 18, "Please Pass the Salt (No, Please *Pass* on the Salt)"
Chapter 21, "Exercise: Get Moving"
Chapter 25, "Weight Loss"
Chapter 26, "Have You Got a Light?: The Perils of Smoking"

5. Reduce your stress level.

Chapter 23, "The Motor's Always Running: Chronic Stress and Your Blood Pressure"

6. Understand the role of complementary and alternative medicine in dealing with your blood pressure.

Chapter 30, "Complementary and Alternative medicine (CAM)"
Chapter 31, "CAM: What Really Works?"
Chapter 34, "CAM: A Realistic and Workable Approach"

7. If lifestyle changes don't get your blood pressure where it needs to be, work with your physician to determine the best medication for you.

Chapter 35, "I've Tried Everything!"
Chapter 36, "Pearls from the Experts"
Chapter 38, "When It Comes to BP Medicines, What Choices Do We Have?"

8. What medicines do we have to choose from, and what are the risks?

Chapter 39, "The Water Pills"

Chapter 41, "The Calcium Channel Blockers (CCBs)"
Chapter 43, "The Beta-Blockers: What They Are and How They Work"
Chapter 45, "Keep an ACE Up Your Sleeve: The ACE Inhibitors"
Chapter 47, "The Angiotensin Receptor Blockers (ARBs): Just Another ACE?"
Chapter 49, "Combination Blood Pressure Drugs: Are They Worth It?"
Chapter 51, "The Big Guns: When All Else Fails"

9. Where do we turn when we need practical, straightforward, and unbiased advice?

Chapter 55, "Don't Be Misled"

10. Monitor your progress. Keep a record of your blood pressure, weight, and blood work.

Chapter 11, "Home Blood Pressure Monitoring: Is It a Waste of Time?"

11. Find the balance in your life. We are all designed to be centered, and that includes our physical health, our emotional lives, and our spiritual being.

Chapter 56, "It's All About Balance"

12. Make a commitment, trust that you will succeed, and let's get started! Remember, "A journey of a thousand miles begins with a single step" (Lao-tzu).

"For I know the plans I have for you,"
declares the LORD,
"plans to prosper you and not to harm you,
plans to give you hope and a future."
(Jeremiah 29:11)

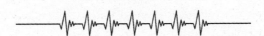

60

You Gotta Know Your Numbers

That's right—you gotta know your numbers. And you gotta put that knowledge to good use.

"Knowledge is not power.
The implementation of knowledge is power."
Larry Winget (1952–)

About the Author

Bestselling author Dr. Robert Lesslie is a physician with more than 30 years of experience working in or directing fast-paced, intense ER environments. He is now the co-owner and medical director of two urgent-care facilities. He has written *60 Ways to Lower Your Cholesterol*, *Notes from a Doctor's Pocket*, *Angels on the Night Shift*, *Angels and Heroes*, *Angels on Call*, *Miracles in the ER*, and *Angels in the ER* (over 200,000 sold) as well as newspaper and magazine columns and human-interest stories. He and his wife, Barbara, live in South Carolina.

You can contact Dr. Lesslie through his blog at http://robert lesslie.com/blog.